PRAISE FOR

tenderheaded

"Because of the variety of voices in *TENDERHEADED* . . . the book has a feeling of breadth and nuance."

—*The Washington Post*

"A must-read that unravels our deep-rooted history and relationship with hair."

—*Heart and Soul*

"Peter Harris' piece . . . is just one gem in this outstanding volume."

—*The Boston Herald*

"Perfectly captures black people's progress (or lack of it) on the hair issue. . . . Valuable and enlightening to anyone who is tenderheaded in one way or another."

—*The Times-Picayune* (New Orleans)

"It's time to get down to the nappy truth about all the pros and cons of black hair. Harris and Johnson's 'comb-bending collection' is a tell-it-like-it-is compilation of essays that give insight into what we and others think about it, the history behind our hair, and how it affects our lives."

—*Black Issues Book Review*

"This remarkable array of writings and images illuminates black women's hair and its cultural meaning. . . . Beyond the variety of contributors and the provocative quotes and historical tidbits sprinkled between the entries, it's the wealth of feeling rooted in hair that makes this volume so compelling. With its (s)nappy jacket and generous helpings of art and photos, this mini-encyclopedia should attract an avid audience."

—*Publishers Weekly*

tenderheaded

A Comb-Bending Collection of Hair Stories

Edited by
Juliette Harris and Pamela Johnson

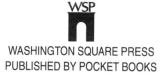

WASHINGTON SQUARE PRESS
PUBLISHED BY POCKET BOOKS

New York   London   Toronto   Sydney   Singapore

"It All Comes Down to the Kitchen," from *Colored People* by Henry Louis Gates Jr. Copyright © 1994 by Henry Louis Gates Jr. Reprinted by permission of Alfred A. Knopf, a division of Random House, Inc.

"Tenderheaded (or Rejecting the Legacy of Being Able to Take It)" by Meg Henson Scales. Copyright © 1995 (although this was copyrighted in 1995, this is its first publication in print media).

"Planet Hair," from *Bulletproof Diva* by Lisa Jones. Copyright © 1994 by Lisa Jones. Used by permission of Doubleday, a division of Random House, Inc.

"Grandma Blows Her Top," from *Pushed Back to Strength* by Gloria Wade-Gayles. Copyright © 1993 by Gloria Wade-Gayles. Reprinted by permission of Beacon Press, Boston.

"Battle of the Wigs," from *The Colored Museum* by George C. Wolfe. Copyright © 1985, 1987, 1988 by George C. Wolfe. Used by permission of Grove/Atlantic, Inc.

Excerpt from *Song of Solomon* by Toni Morrison. Reprinted by permission of International Creative Management, Inc. Copyright © 1977.

"Afro Images: Politics, Fashion and Nostalgia" by Angela Y. Davis, from *Names We Call Home*. Reprinted by permission of Routledge. Copyright © 1996.

"My Smart Grey Streak" by Yvonne Durant. Originally published in *Essence*. Reprinted by permission of the author.

"Homage to My Hair" by Lucille Clifton. First published in *Two Headed Woman*. Copyright © 1980. Originally published by University of Massachusetts Press. Reprinted by permission of Curtis Brown, Ltd.

"She Who Mirrors Me," excerpt from *With Ossie and Ruby: In This Life Together* by Ossie Davis and Ruby Dee. Copyright © 1998 by Ossie Davis and Ruby Dee. Reprinted by permission of HarperCollins Publishers, Inc.

"Clean Break," from *Straight, No Chaser* by Jill Nelson. Copyright © 1997 by Jill Nelson. Used by permission of Putnam Berkley, a division of Penguin Putnam, Inc.

"Oppressed Hair Puts a Ceiling on the Brain" by Alice Walker. From *Living by the Word: Selected Writings 1973–1987*. Printed by permission of Harcourt, Inc. Copyright © 1998.

A Washington Square Press Publication of
POCKET BOOKS, a division of Simon & Schuster, Inc.
1230 Avenue of the Americas, New York, NY 10020

ISBN: 0-671-04756-6

First Washington Square Press trade paperback printing February 2002

10 9 8 7 6 5 4 3 2 1

WASHINGTON SQUARE PRESS and colophon are registered trademarks of Simon & Schuster, Inc.

For information regarding special discounts for bulk purchases, please contact Simon & Schuster Special Sales at 1-800-456-6798 or business@simonandschuster.com

Cover illustration © 1978 by Varnette Honeywood, titled *Dixie Peach*, from the collection of Dr. and Mrs. Rudolph Moragne

Printed in the U.S.A.

This bow is for you. . . .

To Sylvia, Gary and Thai, for all the many reasons why, including welcoming the hair muses and furies into the family and making a generous place for them at the table.

JULIETTE

For the Mamacita, the Papasan and Keren, my beautiful little sister who towers above me. And for women writers everywhere: say it or it won't get said.

PAMELA

Hats off to . . . Diane & LaVon

. . . Our mamas, Olive and Joyce, and black mothers all, for keeping our heads well-greased and pointed in the right direction.

. . . Our contributors, who made us giggle and sniffle and dig deeper into the complexity of our issues than we ever imagined we'd go.

. . . Our agent, Victoria Sanders, who pitched the project like she was throwing fast balls in the World Series. Plus a nod to Selena James, her capable relief pitcher.

. . . Our editor, Greer Kessel Hendricks, a sister of another tribe who, alas, has endured her own tenderheaded times. A tip of the comb as well to her pleasant assistant, Suzanne O'Neill.

. . . Our angels: A'Lelia Bundles, Setaya M. Hodges, Patricia W. Johnson, Linda Jones, Leatha Mitchell, Jenyne Raines, Fo Wilson, and Cherilyn "Liv" Wright, who let us borrow their wings when ours were grounded.

. . . Our Ansisters & our Creator for filling our heads with fanciful ideas and giving us the wooly, wacky hair with which to pull them off.

Ase!

Contents

Ms. Strand Calls a
Press Conference

Our hair speaks with a voice as soft as cotton. If you listen closely—put your ear right up to it—it will tell you its secrets. Like the soothing peace it knew before being yanked out of Africa. Like the neglect it endured sweating under rags in the sun-lashed fields of the South. And even today, it speaks of its restless quest for home; a place that must be somewhere between Africa and America, between rambunctious and restrained, and between personally pleasing and socially "acceptable." For the longest time . . .

Wait a minute. . . . It appears as if . . . Yes, it's Ms. Strand, herself.

A single, slender, crinkly hair makes her way to the stage. She has been through so much trauma that she can sing the "Battle Hymn of the Republic" backward. She's called together her favorite writers to help her tell her story.

"Hello, can you all hear me back there? And you over there? Good. First off, thank you all for coming to my press conference today. I've been meaning to hold one for the longest time, but I got a little tied up, what with slavery, Jim Crow and almost sliding down the drain this morning.

"As you all know, over the centuries, I've been 'buked and I've been scorned, I've been talked about sure as you're born, as the old spiritual goes. Today, though, I'm going to lay my burden down, tell it all. But if I have to do it by myself, it'll take me another 400 years. So I need your help. I need all of you tenderheads here to go deep within yourselves and tell what's in your heart. Don't hold nothing back. I believe we can have a healing in here today.

"Ntozake, you've definitely been through some hair changes and ain't never been afraid to talk about the most painful things, maybe cause you also see the joy, so I need you to start us off. . . ."

Peace Be Still

Ntozake Shange

Peace be still now before we touch my head / we are still / so i can get in this head / not be still before i burn you / be still / so i can get this part straight / be still / i know that didn't hurt / not / be still or this mess is gonna get in your eyes / not be still / fore i pull out the little hair you got / not be still / so i can get in this "kitchen" / not be still / so i can make you pretty / just / be still / then yvette & kim who braid my hair with me / lay on hands / & we feel all the pains and glories that every little nappy strand knows / we let our spirits carry away fear & shame / carry away envy & history / we bless my head

we don't bless out my head / askin' / why did god do this to you chile / even though i could tell from the way my grandma touched my scalp / she loved me / what she was lettin me know / maybe god didn't love me & my brown krinkly short head of hair was a mark / lettin the whole world know / god's not on this chile's side / god has marked her / as toomer said / "oh can't you see it / oh can't you see it" / her hair is cursed from the western horizon / oh can't you see it / & then everything turns back on itself / literally / the beauty shop smells are com- forting / dixie peach melting on hot curlin' irons delicious / mirrors are a source of pleasure / who says colored girls aren't pretty / look at me now miz harshaw's worked her magic / not a nap to be found / not one hair to curl up under itself like a slinky / now straight / & makin' me precious in the sight of god

anything / you can do to your hair / i do believe i've done it / looking for grace & my crazed notion that i'd be the kinda girl my daddy'd like to marry if my hair was better / but the bad hair came from his side of the family / & how does that make me feel about my own flesh & blood / when i was very little / my parents had a grand fete & for some reason god had blessed all the women & most of the men with good hair / not that my hair wasn't done / mommy'd gotten us up early to get our heads out the way / but her straightening comb wasn't deluxe like miz harshaw's & sometimes it slipped a lil just behind my ears / but that's not the story / all the guests had fresh towels out on their beds / i know cuz i put em there / but i'd seen carmen delavallade and dorothy dandridge too / they had the blessings / i wrapped my head in one of the bath towels / of one of god's sacred ladies / & did something of a chile follows katherine dunham to ecstasy / contract & plié / turn turn turn turn leap / fall to knees spin torso / shake shake shake / relevé / and jump / pose with arms extended / back arch / and relax / fully expectin' / this ritual to bless me now that i'd been able to let him know what i hankered after / the blessing / the glory of god fallen round my shoulders just like the towel / we know / that didn't happen / but i was shocked & settled for dusting my face with talcum powder / i was gonna get on god's good side one way or another /

skip years / skip short cropped afros / slicked gel on twiggy pixie looks / skip page boys / skip not learnin how to swim cuz my hair'd turn back / skip lookin at me after a boisterous dance in the summer's heat of night / skip livin' with not bein' beauteous in god's eyes for most of my life / till my friends said / be still / let the spirits come / & we braid / we braid / we twist / & we braid / some of us straighten and curl / or leave the curls to wind in the wind / and then maybe finger curl or loop the hair around our necks and wait for the glory that is ours to transform itself to geometric glittering shapes befitting nefertiti or ropey loops like sally hemmings / we are tossed all colors known to man / some krinkly some wavy / some straighter n straight / but we have that moment now among friends to glance at our varied heads of hair and sigh / peace be still

—*ntozake shange, houston, april 2000*

Heads of Steam

here we celebrate the pioneering women who taught us how to smooth the kinks in our hair, as well as those frontier mamas who brought us back to the bush.

WHY COLORED FOLKS HAVE NAPPY HAIR —A FOLKTALE

In the beginning, the story goes, nobody had hair. So God called everybody together to beautify them and hand out the hair. When the call came that the hair was ready, black folks were having a big barbeque that they wanted to finish. The other races came running, put the hair on, and smoothed it down. And so they have smooth hair. Then they issued a second call to the colored people. But the only hair that was left was the trampled hair on the ground. So the colored folks got stuck with the kinky hair.

RUNAWAY SLAVES WITH FLYAWAY HAIR

Eighteenth-century advertisements for runaway slaves described numerous unruly hair styles like the one worn by "Hannah," who, according to an ad, had "her Hair . . . lately cut in a very irregular Manner, as a Punishment for Offences."

IN OTHER WORDS . . .

GOOD HAIR: Back in the day (and some still believe), a close approximation of Caucasian hair. The texture is generally wavy and silky soft to the touch. Of course, the length is long, or the hair has the potential to be long. Some folks used to call it "nearer-my-God-to-thee hair."

BAD HAIR: Tightly coiled, "coarse" hair that is thought to be hard to "manage" and is generally short. Also known as nappy hair, tight hair, and <u>mailman hair, as in "every knot's got its own route."</u>

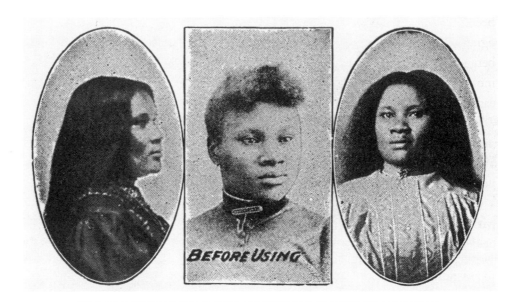

Madam C. J. Walker (pictured here) was a pioneer in modern advertising and marketing techniques. According to A'Lelia Bundles, the "after" photographs are not doctored.

A'LELIA BUNDLES/WALKER FAMILY COLLECTION

MADAM C. J. WALKER: "LET ME CORRECT THE ERRONEOUS IMPRESSION THAT I CLAIM TO STRAIGHTEN HAIR"
A'Lelia Bundles

Whitfield's official title may have been janitor of the Mme C. J. Walker Manufacturing Company, but I still think of him as the Indiana Avenue ambassador who greeted my mother and me whenever we arrived at the block-long brick headquarters in her 1955 black Mercury.

Once inside the foyer, I was always fascinated by Mary Martin's shiny, finger-waved tresses and cherry-rouged cheeks as she snapped shut the accordion brass elevator gate with one fluid flick of her wrist, then lifted us four floors toward my mother's office. Another glissade of Mary's manicured hands and the percussive clickity-clack of my mother's spike heels led me across a cayenne-flecked marble terrazzo lobby.

With each step—first past Mrs. Overstreet, the bookkeeper who would have been a CPA had she been born sixty years later, then past Edith Shanklin, the address-ograph operator who always had a gossip morsel for my mother—the syrupy aroma of bergamot and Glossine from the factory downstairs made me wish for candy. In my mother's office a hand-cranked adding machine and manual typewriter awaited my eager fingers.

Throughout my childhood, my mother, A'Lelia Mae Perry Bundles, was vice president of the hair care and cosmetics firm founded by Madam Walker in 1906. By a twist of fate, my grandmother, Mae, whose silky braids roped below her waist, was legally adopted by Madam Walker's daughter, A'Lelia Walker. As a walking advertisement for "Walker's Wonderful Hair Grower," Mae traveled with Madam Walker as a model, was entrusted with the "secret" formulas, then became president of the Walker Company after A'Lelia Walker's death in 1931.

Early in my parents' marriage, my father, S. Henry Bundles, had been a salesman for Apex, another black hair-care company, then became general sales manager of the Walker Company for a few years during the mid-1950s.

More comfortable with the notion of making his own way despite the impressive history of his wife's family's company, he accepted an offer to become president of Summit Laboratories—one of the then-new generation of black hair-care companies that had modern marketing ideas, chemical straighteners, and aggressive sales forces.

Growing up in a household where hair-care products put food on the table meant that the weekly kitchen-counter hair-washing ritual assumed meaning beyond just what happened between Momma, me, and the thick-toothed, ebony shampoo comb. Even some family vacations were dictated by the time and locale of the summer hair-industry conventions; I was fascinated by their flamboyant stylists and fantasy coiffure extravaganzas. As a teenager I knew the names of all the inner-city beauty and barber supply houses from Harlem to Oakland because my first non-baby-sitting job was filing their invoices and order forms in my father's office.

My father's work at Summit Laboratories allowed a comfortable life for us, provided the occasional Caribbean vacation, and sent me to college. And though the Walker Company's influence was dwindling by the early 1960s, it was the pioneering efforts of Madam Walker and some of her contemporaries that had created the climate for Summit and dozens of other firms in the now $3-billion-a-year ethnic hair-care market.

Throughout my childhood, I had heard Madam Walker's almost mythical, rags-to-riches litany often enough to memorize it: born Sarah Breedlove in 1867, she was orphaned at seven, married at fourteen, a mother at seventeen, widowed at twenty. She worked as a washerwoman until she began to go bald. Miraculously, she claimed, the scalp treatment that restored her hair and made her wealthy was revealed to her in a dream. When she died in 1919 at fifty-one, she had created the role of a self-made American woman entrepreneur and philanthropist.

In some versions of her story, a "big African man" came to her and told her what to mix up. In others, a pharmacist helped her replicate one of the many scalp ointments already on the market. In still another, Poro founder Annie Malone, one of her fiercest competitors, claimed she stole the formula.

In pursuit of the truth—not just about her formula, but about her life—I have spent more than two decades worth of vacations, leaves, and weekends visiting courthouses, archives, and the living rooms of a most fascinating array of octo- and nonagenarian Walker Company employees, friends, and confidants.

And still, I have questions. Some days I mine a nugget so bright, so clear, that I believe I finally have unlocked her deepest secrets. Other days, I hit a wall so impenetrable that I am overwhelmed.

While I was writing the first major biography about her *(Madam C. J. Walker—A Family Legacy* [Scribner, 2001]), I often found myself speaking to her, asking questions, writing letters. In my imagination, she heard me.

Dear Great-great-grandmother Walker,

As I write this letter, I am surrounded by a wall full of your photographs and files stuffed with hundreds of your letters, newspaper clippings and advertisements.

By the time I was born in 1952, you'd been gone for more than thirty years. But you were not forgotten in our household.

We ate our Thanksgiving turkey on your hand-painted Limoges china and ladled Christmas eggnog from your sterling punch bowl. Great-grandmother A'Lelia's mahogany Chickering baby grand was the focal point of our living room. And treasures from Villa Lewaro, your mansion in Irvington-on-Hudson, New York, accented shelves and tables throughout our house.

At PaPa Perry's—he married A'Lelia's daughter Mae in 1927—I explored your old brown leather trunk, each new compartment more breathtaking than the last. A small lacquered compact of Mme C. J. Walker's Egyptian Tan Powder was tucked near a monogrammed silver-and-tortoiseshell comb. Miniature enameled mummy charms from A'Lelia's 1921 trip to Cairo were stashed next to a gold-tasseled dance card from your 1914 spring musicale featuring Noble Sissle.

One nook overflowed with faded letters and photographs of dignified ebony faces. As I opened a silk-covered drawer, scented, satin lingerie and a musty ostrich feather fan danced with my senses. But it was only years later that I began to fully grasp the legacy those mementos represented.

During the late 1960s while I was in high school, the civil rights movement—something you would have welcomed after your years of support for the NAACP's anti-lynching campaign—was evolving into the Black Power movement and a resurgent interest in black history. The same sense of adventure and anticipation that had led me to your trunk accompanied me through libraries and tattered books in search of knowledge about African Americans. Imagine how my heart raced with the thrill of personal affirmation when the indexes of those dusty volumes revealed not only your name, but A'Lelia Walker's name—my name.

Your former secretary, Violet Reynolds, who was our neighbor, once told me that your relationship with A'Lelia was "like fire and ice. They loved each other deeply and they sometimes fought fiercely."

It was clear from the letter that you wrote to A'Lelia just before you died in May 1919, that you loved spoiling her. It was also clear that she tried very, very hard to please you. You must have known that no matter how strong-willed she was, she never stopped being dependent on you. It was hard for her to measure up to your expectations while you were living, and even harder when everyone made the inevitable comparisons between the two of you.

After you died, she was devastated. And the rest of her life she was never fully freed from the need to satisfy you. But the 1920s were designed perfectly for her, providing a niche in the high-living music and cultural scene of the Harlem Renaissance, at least for a while, for one of the world's first black heiresses. I suspect you wouldn't have approved of her late nights and party-girl reputation, but many people say she was the *essence of the era's flamboyance. She did continue to manage the Walker salon and office that she had persuaded you to establish in New York. If nothing else, she kept your name in the headlines with her lavish soirees.*

I hope you will understand when I tell you that I had some ambivalence about you during the 1960s when so many of us were transforming our hair from perms to naturals. Buoyed by the liberation rhetoric of the times, many people invoked your name as the villain who pushed hair straightening and hot combs. I just wish I'd known what I know now. But it was years before I could verify that you were not the inventor of the straightening comb, and years before I would find the newspaper clipping where you'd told a reporter: "Let me correct the erroneous impression held by some that I claim to straighten hair. I want the great masses of my people to take a greater pride in their appearance and to give their hair proper attention."

Maybe you said that because you were sick of seeing those headlines in the white newspapers: "De-Kink Queen Builds Mansion" or "Negress Makes Millions on Anti-Kink Hair Oil." Or maybe you were trying to distinguish yourself from the companies that denigrated black women with their insulting ads for products guaranteed to "cure ugly skin and bad hair."

Maybe that's why you put your own photograph—the one where your hair bushed out into a long, full mane—on your products. Given the times, that must have been an act of defiance, a declaration that you dared to see yourself as beautiful, a proclamation to other black women that they could have confidence in themselves just as they were.

How was I to know that E. Franklin Frazier—the venerable Howard University sociologist—had gotten it wrong in Black Bourgeoisie *when he accused you of running advertisements that tell how the Negro can rid himself of his black or dark complexion, or how he can straighten his hair: "It was through the manufacture of such products that Madame Walker, one of the first 'rich Negroes' to gain notoriety, made a fortune and set a standard for conspicuous consumption that has become legendary!"*

His words embarrassed me, to tell you the truth. And, at the time, I had no documentation to counter his indictment. I couldn't reconcile his contempt with the other things I was learning about you. But deep down inside I knew you were too much of a race woman to have placed the imitation of whites at the top of your list of priorities.

After another decade of research I learned that while you were alive the Mme C. J. Walker Manufacturing Company never sold skin bleaches, and that you insisted on calling yourself a scalp specialist and hair culturist, never allowing the words "hair straightener" to creep into your ads.

I still don't know where the rumor started that you invented the straightening comb. There's no question that you and scores of other hairdressers popularized its use and that you sold it as part of your kit. But Bloomingdale's, with a presumably mostly white clientele, was selling a metal hot comb called Dr. Scott's Electric Curler as early as 1886 while you were still picking cotton in Mississippi.

It's hard for people to stop believing this hot comb story because it's something they've heard all their lives. Surely their mothers and grandmothers and all the books they've read can't be wrong, they must think.

Still I keep trying to tell them that you were more concerned with baldness than nappiness, that you suffered from a scalp disease called alopecia, caused by poor hygiene, stress, and an unhealthy diet. A lot of folks just can't fathom the severity of the scalp ailments that existed in the early twentieth century. But considering that many women washed their hair only once a month—and even less during the winter—it's no wonder that dandruff and tetter were so bad that pus and blood oozed from some people's scalps. It's a wonder that they had any hair at all.

And yet I know you must have wrestled with the straight versus natural issue. Surely you were not entirely free of the pressure to assimilate in a society that valued Caucasian beauty. But you were much more visionary than you possibly could have realized when you predicted, "I dare say that in the next ten years it will be a rare thing to see a kinky head of hair and it will not be straight either."

It took a few decades longer than you expected, but I think you'd be pleased with the range of styles black women now choose. I recently read somewhere that 75 percent of African-American women straighten their hair either with chemicals, hot combs, rollers, or blow dryers. But since the 1960s, traditional African styles (braids, cornrows, locks, and twists) have remained popular, and most women—regardless of the styles they wear—have adopted the healthier grooming regimen you had hoped they would. Today many women feel free to change their style at will.

But hair still is a very emotional, even political, issue in our community, loaded with centuries of complicated psychological and sociological, well, kinks and tangles. It's often volatile enough to provoke a fight, a lawsuit, or feelings of shame. That lots of people still talk about "good hair" and "bad hair," I think, would make you unhappy.

Women still get fired from their jobs and ostracized because they choose to let their African roots push through. Many men are still way too enamored of long, flowing hair. And deeper than that, there are far too many grown women still smarting from traumatic childhood memories of a mother's disdain for their hard-to-comb hair.

Personally, I must admit that I punt the whole issue and wear my hair short—at least for now—because I'm just too busy to worry about it. And I suspect that this was part of A'Lelia Walker's reason for sporting those beautiful turbans she favored.

Still, I've had people ask me what you would say about my closely cut curls. In some ways, I wonder why anyone would be at all concerned about my hair. But because I was taught to be polite to strangers—and who else but a stranger would ask such a question?—I just tell them that you were a businesswoman, not the hair police, and would have insisted that I use your shampoo rather than someone else's.

When it all comes down to it, I think you were urging women—especially those in the great migration wave from the South to the industrial cities of the North—to improve their appearance so that they could increase their earning power. After a point, I think you became more interested in your ability to create jobs and economic independence for others than you ever were in making money just for yourself. These days it's rare that I make a speech about you when someone doesn't tell me a story about an aunt, a grandmother, or a neighbor whose earnings from hairdressing made a difference in their lives.

I hope you'll understand the decision of the Walker estate trustees to sell the company in 1985. The industry was changing rapidly, all the original trustees had died, and most of the others were nearing retirement. Experts who study family businesses have learned that it's fairly common for the third and fourth generations to pursue other interests. Thankfully my parents understood this. All my life they encouraged me to follow my own dreams—just as you had followed yours. Fortunately I was able to spend more than twenty years as a television news producer for two of the most successful television news organizations in the world, then as a deputy bureau chief for one of them.

As a result, when I made the decision to write your biography, I didn't mind at all that I had come full circle to you—now on my own terms—and that I'm able to use all the professional skills I have learned to tell your story.

Next time I'll tell you about television. (You would have loved the advertising opportunities.) But for now, just know that learning your life is a challenge and a blessing.

With love,
A'Lelia

HOW GREAT WAS SHE?

- In a letter to Madam C. J. Walker, former First Lady Mrs. Grover Cleveland said, "You have opened up a trade for hundreds of colored women to make an honest and profitable living where they make as much in one week as a month's salary would bring from any other position that a colored woman can secure."
- Former maids, washerwomen, cooks, and field workers eagerly reported how they were buying real estate, educating their children and contributing to their churches at the 1917 convention of Madam Walker sales agents and beauty culturists in Philadelphia.
- In the early twentieth century, when $1,000 was a considerable sum, Walker's $1,000 contribution to the building fund of the black YMCA in

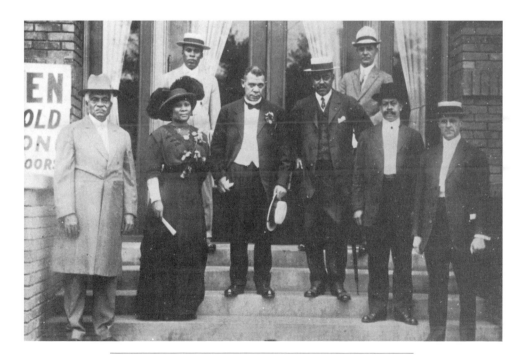

Madam C. J. Walker with Booker T. Walker (man holding hat) and other
black leaders at the dedication of the Senate Avenue YMCA in Indianapolis in 1913.

MADAM C. J. WALKER COLLECTION/INDIANA HISTORICAL SOCIETY

1911 in Indianapolis was an incentive for others to give. Her $5,000 dona-
tion to the NAACP's anti-lynching fund in 1919 was the largest the organization had ever received.

- Walker supported the Silent Protest Parade against the East St. Louis riots
in 1917, and she was part of a delegation that went to the White House to
persuade President Woodrow Wilson to support anti-lynching legislation.
She also argued for the civil rights of black World War I soldiers and vet-
erans.

- There are two National Historic Landmarks associated with Walker: Villa
Lewaro in Irvington-on-Hudson, New York, and the Madam Walker Theatre Center in Indianapolis, where the Walker Company was based from
1927 through 1985.

- In 1998 Walker joined her friends Mary McLeod Bethune, W. E. B. Du
Bois, James Weldon Johnson, Booker T. Washington, A. Philip Randolph,
and Ida B. Wells-Barnett when she became the twenty-first subject of the
U.S. Postal Service's Black Heritage Series.

- Walker was named a "20th Century Builder and Titan" in a special issue of
Time magazine.

WE'VE KNOWN RIVERS

Settling near rivers, streams, and other plentiful water sources, West African
women developed important deities, like the river spirit, Yemanja, and communal
beauty rituals associated with water and cleanliness. On the American plantation,
however, there was little or no access to flowing waters. In an oral account, a former enslaved black man recalls that the communal aspect of grooming continued
in slavery but without the benefits of flowing water:

> On Sundays the old folks stayed home and looked one another's
> heads over for nits and lice. Whenever they found anything, they mashed
> it twixt they finger and thumb and went ahead searching. Then the
> women wrapped each other's hair the way it was to stay fixed till the next
> Sunday.

THE HAIRDRESSER AND THE SCHOLAR
Mark Higbee

In 1937 Benjamin Stolberg, a white writer, denounced Madam C. J. Walker's "hair unkinking process" as an insult to the racial integrity of black people. W. E. B. Du Bois, the great African-American thinker and political leader, came to Madam Walker's defense, contending that Stolberg's charge against the hair-care pioneer was oversimplified. This little-known squabble over race, hair, and identity had surfaced before and would come up again and again in African-American life.

In the 1920s, back-to-Africa movement founder Marcus Garvey held views like those later expressed by Stolberg. Again differing from his rival, Du Bois, Garvey denounced hair straightening as an affront to race pride. Few were listening. Even in his own camp, ads for hair-straightening products, which many Garveyite women used, continued to be published in Garvey's *Negro World* newspaper.

• 1914 •

In his book *Social Ethics*, J. M. Mecklin, a white writer, maintains that the new hair-straightening convention shows that black folks lack pride.

In the 1960s the argument resurfaced as proponents of "black consciousness" argued that the African-American hair-care industry promoted white ideals of beauty. These values, they asserted, were then internalized by black people. Indeed, as early as 1962 the future Black Panther leader Eldridge Cleaver blasted the black beauty industry and its customers in an article, "As Crinkly as Yours, Brother," for the Nation of Islam's newspaper, which was then known as *Muhammad Speaks*.

While most prominent blacks who have spoken out on this issue have focused their discussions on physical and psychological factors, Du Bois saw those arguments as shortsighted. Madam C. J. Walker's business was "epoch-making," Du Bois wrote on the occasion of her death in 1919, both for what it did to create the African-American beauty industry and for its other economic contributions to "the race." His *Crisis* magazine obituary for Walker praised her as "A Great Woman" who had "transform[ed] a people in a generation."

Walker's leading-edge instincts stemmed from her understanding that, in the years following emancipation, African-American women needed to reinvent themselves. Coming of age during those transitional years, Walker discerned that

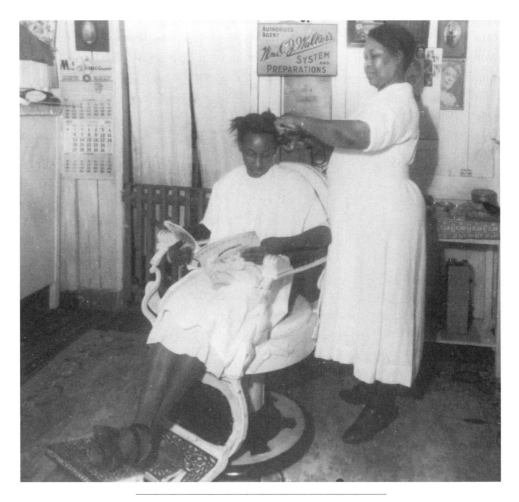

Authorized Walker System agent smoothing those nappy edges.

A'LELIA BUNDLES/WALKER FAMILY COLLECTION

hair and dress were central to black women's declaration of independence: The headrags and hand-me-downs of their enslavement were simply not appropriate for their new lives as free women. Du Bois recognized the breadth of Walker's vision and praised her achievements as an important contribution to black womanhood.

In 1937, as the employment crisis of the Great Depression deepened, Du Bois specifically praised the Walker Company for creating "perhaps 13,000 jobs" for black women, making them "almost independent entrepreneurs." Walker had established her business by traveling around the country, personally recruiting women into her nationwide brigade of beauty-culture agents. They all learned the Walker system of pressing hair and selling her products.

Interestingly, the claim that Walker's products were an "anthropological insult" to black people—the criticism leveled in *The Nation* magazine by Stolberg, an independent Marxist writer, and by Garvey and later Cleaver—consistently came from the mouths of males. In each case, they interpreted African-American women's choices as evidence of racial self-hatred. Neither Cleaver nor Stolberg nor Garvey considered that black women had their own distinct ideas of beauty, shaped by their personal experience and by their gender.

Writing in the *Pittsburgh Courier* (then the nation's leading black weekly) in December 1937, Du Bois argued that "it is no more an 'anthropological insult' for one person to have hair straightened than for another to have his hair curled." Fashion was fashion and style was style, not self-hatred, he reasoned.

When the consumer age was just dawning in the early 1900s, Walker became a marketing pioneer by using her image to sell her products. And she projected that image forcefully: a hardworking but glamorous colored woman who had pulled herself up from the cotton fields and washtubs to become a "millionaire." Madam C. J. Walker's story sat well both with America's pro-business ideology and with the aspirations of African-American women to be stylish, beautiful, and independent, all on terms defined by themselves, not by whites or men.

Although Du Bois greatly admired Walker and praised her company, in the 1930s he was highly critical of African-American business, in general, for failing to use its "tremendous power" to transform the condition of all black people, not just the entrepreneurial class. In 1937 he applied this broad criticism to the Walker Company as well. He envisioned the small businesses run by Walker agents and other black women as a network that could become part of the foundation for a strong, independent black nation within the nation, and, in a truly revolutionary turn, marry small business enterprises with a socialist system. The latter would provide for the material needs of all African Americans, Du Bois asserted: "A little broader knowledge and far-seeing advice might easily have turned the Walker hair culture business during her [Walker's] life into a co-operative enterprise and this co-operation, instead of being a group capitalistic movement could have been given the form of a socialistic mass movement, not only in hair culture but other lines. What is true of the Walker business can be true of the whole inner economic organization of American Negroes."

Had Madam C. J. Walker, who died at fifty-one in 1919, lived longer, she might have pursued some version of this race-based economic program. In her last years, in fact, she became a staunch political activist. She joined anti-lynching crusades and was one of eleven blacks who planned to hold a protest meeting outside the 1919 peace conference in Versailles, France. This protest, organized by fiery civil rights advocate William Monroe Trotter, aimed to demand equal rights for black people in America and in Europe's African colonies. Walker supported Trotter, despite the advice of her business manager, who warned that her political activities could harm her business. But the Trotter group's plans were foiled when the State Department denied them visas.

Walker and Du Bois, given time, might also have worked together for common political goals. Perhaps then, in 1937, instead of taking the company to task, Du Bois might have persuaded Walker to join him in pushing his plan for African-American economic development. The hairdresser and the scholar would have made quite a team!

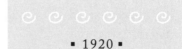

▪ 1920 ▪

W. E. B. Du Bois poetically blesses black women's kinky heads in the essay "The Damnation of Women," in *Darkwater:* if a woman is "pink and white and straight-haired, and some of her fellow-men prefer this, well and good; but if she is black or brown and crowned in curled mists (and this to us is the most beautiful thing on earth), this is surely the flimsiest excuse for spiritual incarceration or banishment."

HOW TIGHT IS IT?

The teeny-tiny circumferences of kinks have been described as:

b.b.s
beadabees
peas
peazy head
snap-back knots

SEVERED

Annabelle Baker

It was 1943, my second year at Hampton Institute, and the second year that the world was at war. I remember the times for the sense of urgency that gripped the nation. We could even feel it on our beautiful waterfront campus in Virginia, where I was an honor student. My major was art and English education, and I wrote profiles of notable people on campus in a column for the *Hampton Script* called "Personality at a Glance."

Some of the buildings on campus were used exclusively by the navy, which meant a new group of Negro sailors, fresh out of boot camp, arriving every few weeks. Those sailors who were departing seemed to strut, buoyed by their new ranks and the tears and promises of Hampton's co-eds.

We students did our part for the cause by forgoing meat on Thursdays, even as we smelled the savory roasts and chops from the adjoining navy dining room. We all hated what we called "meatless Thursdays"! Looking back, however, I'd have to say it was a minor sacrifice. I was so happy at Hampton. I felt so alive and hungry to learn. I remember bonding closely with the art students there. We were encouraged by Professor Victor Lowenfeld's guidance to "paint what you know," even as most students criticized paintings that depicted scenes of black life.

This immersion into art led me on a personal quest to understand and define "art" and "beauty." I concluded that art or beauty was "the thing unto itself." To appreciate that beauty was to be able to look with eyes unclouded by preconceptions and prejudices; to be able to listen without filtering what one hears through one's own opinions; and to be able to learn without interjecting what one thinks one knows. In doing this, we have encountered "the thing unto itself." I think that's what Gertrude Stein meant when she said, "A rose is a rose is a rose."

Coming to regard nature as the perfect artist, I was enchanted by her use of line, color, texture, and even "theme." As I began to look differently at the human form, developing a new regard for bone structure, skin tone, and hair texture, I began to see the whole spectrum of black people as beautiful—not just the "fair to middling" part. In honor of this growing appreciation, I decided to wear my hair natural. One day I left my dorm room and walked a short distance to a small barbershop near campus. I told the lone barber there that I wanted my hair washed but not straightened. I described the shape of the cut I wanted to him: a short bob with a part on the right side.

The slightly built, graying man understood me perfectly. As he put the scissors down, I regarded my "natural" bob as beautiful. Though this was a good twenty-five years before the Afro came into vogue for black women, going natural seemed a simple step to me at the time. But it changed my life forever.

When I reached campus, some students regarded me with complete shock, others with curiosity, and still more with outright hostility. Most of the arguments took place in the dormitory. Even those students who accepted me never raised their voices to defend me. I felt alone. The moment ushered in an excruciatingly painful period in my life. I was so young and immature, and I didn't know where to put the pain. So for many years, I hid it in a bottle.

Try as I might, I couldn't understand how my choice about my head had caused so much furor. But now, as I reflect back more than fifty years, I have concluded that many of the students were battling secret feelings of racial inferiority. By rejecting ourselves in our natural, unaltered state, we were unknowingly perpetuating those feelings.

For me, hair has always been a subject fraught with trouble. In my early childhood, Grandma would section my hair into neat square parts, grease my scalp with Excellenta pomade, and plait the hair, always carefully incorporating the ends of the previous plait into the next one. I hated this grooming routine. I was made to sit still for too long, rigidly holding my head in uncomfortable positions, for results that hardly seemed worth all the effort.

The *number* of plaits Grandma gave me held social significance. The fewer the braids, the greater the social event I was being readied for. Multiple plaits were for casual times like sleeping or staying around the house. Three large plaits—one on top and two side by side below, were for school or church. For really special occasions, like Easter, I wore no plaits at all. At those times, my hair would be straightened with a hot comb and the ends turned up with a curling iron. These heavy metal tools had the power to make me feel pretty or, when they accidently touched my skin, to inflict pain.

By the time I'd reached kindergarten, around 1929, most black children had realized, in their own way, that their hair texture either added to or diminished their social status. Having digested the concepts of "good hair" and "bad hair," we knew in advance who would be the prince or princess or madonna in the school or church dramas. Usually the lighter-complexioned, straighter-haired children won the lead roles. The other parts were then graded down in importance, until finally antagonistic or clownish characters were assigned to the darkest children.

I graduated from plaits around thirteen years old, and was allowed to go to the beautician every two weeks. She knew to give me only a soft press and a few curls. Between visits, I was forbidden to use hot combs or curlers. Meanwhile, I watched as the women in my family touched up their own hair. I didn't see anything drastic happening to them, so when they were at work, I began touching up my own hair. This practice came to a halt one morning when I saw a chunk of my hair remain on the curlers, even as I pulled them away from my head. I had burned off a lot of hair. Luckily, my fear and panic combined to create some rather nice bangs. That evening when the family noticed my new look, I lied and said I had chosen a style like Claudette Colbert's.

I was a world away from those warm feelings of love and acceptance as the end of the '43 school term drew near. Sitting on a bench on campus, wearing my new hairstyle and feeling dejected, I was surprised when a German math professor approached me and asked if I would be interested in attending a two-week, all-expense-paid conference at Wellesley College in Springfield, Massachusetts. She told me that the event's sponsor had decided to invite undergraduates and instructors from different regions of the country. She said she'd selected me, though I'd never been in her class, because she considered me an achiever. I'd never heard of Wellesley, but her offer lifted my spirits.

When Flemmie P. Kittrell, dean of women at Hampton, learned that I'd been selected, she was furious. She thought my hair made me unsuitable to represent the college. But the math professor, whose name I can no longer recall, defied Kittrell and would not surrender her authority to make the selection. Kittrell would not concede, either. She said unchaperoned student travel was not allowed. That requirement was satisfied when I found out that Miss Hunt, matron of Virginia Cleveland Hall, one of the campus dorms, was going by train in my same direction.

Dean Kittrell, whose influence had grown from one small office to almost half of the main floor of the administration building, redoubled her efforts. She called a meeting of deans and administrators for the sole purpose of preventing me from attending the conference. Though I was not allowed to attend the meeting, Professor Lowenfeld spoke up on my behalf. Afterward he told me about the meeting. A recent Jewish immigrant from Austria whose English was not fluent, he relayed to me that he had initially floundered in his attempts to find the words to describe the beauty of my hair. But during the meeting his eyes happened to fall on Miss Hunt, who was seated beneath one of the windows of the Academy Building, the sun pouring through the tall, unshaded window directly onto her hair. In preparation for her trip, she had gotten it hard pressed and tightly curled. The sun's heat melted the oil in her hair and made it run down her face. Seeing that, Professor Lowenfeld said, gave him the sudden inspiration he needed to offer an impassioned plea about how much more beautiful natural hair is than hair that is fried with grease running down it. I don't know how he did it, but somehow he won my permission to go to Wellesley.

In retrospect, I realize that Dean Kittrell was under a lot of pressure. She knew that, as Negro students, we were judged not only for what was in our heads but also for how we presented ourselves. An impressive role model (she was the first African-American woman to earn a Ph.D. in home economics when she graduated from Cornell in 1937), Kittrell wanted Hampton's young ladies to also go out into the world as standard-bearers of deportment and achievement.

At Wellesley, I did my best to conduct myself in a way that upheld Hampton's high standards. I was awed by the many speakers of international prominence, as well as by the school's grand halls and grounds. Everything was wonderful until shortly after I returned to my room one night. That's when I heard a tapping at my door. Outside were two strikingly beautiful Negro co-eds visiting from another prestigious, predominantly white college. Each was well dressed, with hair that flowed into long page boys. They told me that they had come to talk to me about my hair, and they were not smiling. As they entered my room, they told me that I should be ashamed to be seen with my hair in its natural state. I dismissed them quickly and tried to recapture the happiness I felt before they'd come.

My enthusiasm remained high as I attended the closing sessions of the conference, taking copious notes. Students who participated in important off-campus activities were usually asked to make a report about their trips in a student assembly. But when I returned to campus, nobody asked me to give a report.

Going back to school for my junior year did not provide the refuge that I'd hoped for. I was suspended in the first semester for breaking a rule that I didn't know existed; there had been a slight change in the student handbook regarding absenteeism and class-cutting. It was my fault that I didn't read up on it, but still, I felt that the administration had been lying in ambush for me, especially since I was the only student that year suspended under that ruling. Besides, nearly all of my class absences that term were with prior approval of the professors, and with extra asignments to make up for the time lost. Was it me, I wondered, or was it the hair?

I spent the first suspension period right across the water in Norfolk, Virginia, where the Young family, owners and publishers of the *Norfolk Journal and Guide,* gave me a job rewriting copy. During that time I sketched a picture of my predicament. Professor Lowenfeld was impressed with the work and awarded me a $300 scholarship, which was more than enough to cover costs for the term.

Things were looking up until I got myself suspended during the second semester. Though I'd made the honor roll, my absence from classes put me in violation again. I'm surprised more art students weren't punished, since, at the art center, we didn't follow regular hours and many of us practically lived there. When I was not painting, I was working in the sculpture and ceramics area, and often lost track of time.

With the second suspension, I retreated home to Jacksonville. I was embarrassed not only about being expelled twice but also about the shame that my hairstyle caused my family. My hair was a particular affront to my aunts, who cared for me in the wake of my mother's and grandmother's deaths, because they ran the largest beauty parlor in Jacksonville! The pressure eventually became unbearable. Finally, I moved out and found acceptance among the illiterate or minimally educated working class. It was with this group that I began to drink.

The alcohol only intensified the immense loneliness I'd always felt. There was the trauma of being abandoned by my natural mother when I was an infant and my sister was three. We lived near a main street in St. Petersburg, Florida, and my sister would wander, picking up scraps from the ground to eat. One day, the authorities followed her home and found me alone and emaciated. I was taken to Mercy Hospital in St. Petersburg but was not expected to live. At the hospital, one nurse adopted my sister; another adopted me. She is the only mother I have ever known, and we became very close.

Although she was kind to me and my aunts were generous, a huge gulf remained in my life—always shadowing me, threatening to swallow me whole. The gulf deepened when I was twelve years old and my second mother died unexpectedly.

During the summer after the second suspension, I returned from Jacksonville to Hampton, took a room in town, and got a job as a waitress in the Chamberlin Hotel. With tips the pay was fair, but it didn't take long to realize that I would not earn enough money to return to school in September. What made matters worse is that I had not stopped drinking.

One day Dr. Margaret Altman, head of the Department of Agriculture, saw me walking with one of my paintings. My despair must have been apparent. I imagine she noticed my borderline delirium tremens. I felt so lost: my class had graduated, Professor Lowenfeld had taken a position at Penn State, and I didn't like the new professor of art because he wasn't Professor Lowenfeld.

That day, as I told Dr. Altman about my situation, she offered to finance my coming year at Hampton. She also bought me clothes and ended up paying for a summer intercession as well, so I could complete the credits I needed to graduate. All she asked was that I stop drinking. But I couldn't.

One day Dr. Altman, who always looked like a Prussian general (but who was extraordinarily gentle underneath), decided enough was enough. She had helped me, and I had let her down. I had to grow up, and I chose to go to New York to do it. I thought I might find myself there. Also the modern dancer Pearl Primus (who also wore her hair natural) had visited the art center, bought one of my paintings, and suggested I visit if ever I made it to New York.

Dr. Altman drove me to the train station and bought me a one-way ticket. In New York I stayed temporarily in Primus's Eighth Avenue studio. I still called Dr. Altman from time to time for a dose of mothering. "You've got to do something for somebody else," she would admonish me. At the time that made no sense to me, since I was struggling so hard for my own survival.

I didn't understand her advice until years later when a woman that I had known for thirty years as a friend and lover developed a brain tumor. I wanted to help her, but drinking was getting in my way. Finally I had the motivation to quit drinking for good.

In 1971, at forty-six years old, I completed a one-year course in practical nursing. From then until my retirement in 1991, I was a very good nurse, and I still volunteer as a health advocate. But the pain of those earlier years is still real for me—and not all of it was caused by others. A large part of it is the regret and sorrow I feel for disappointing so many friends over the years. Some are gone, and aren't around for me to offer my apologies. But I will never be sorry that I wore my hair natural.

HOT COMB, COOL SOLUTION

In the early 1940s, Billie Holiday worked at Kelly's Stable on New York City's Fifty-Second Street—a.k.a. "Swing Street." One night the house band sounded just like the tune they were playing, "Sweet and Mellow." Lady Day, about to go on, was grooving to the music through the cracked door of her tiny dressing room. She loosened up her throat with a swig of gin and a tote of one of them funny cigarettes. Sylvia Sims, an aspiring singer from Brooklyn, sat in the corner watching her idol with adoration. Nodding her head to the beat, Lady grabbed a curling iron off the Sterno and turned her shoulder-length hair under. Getting lost in the time of the tune, she kept the iron sizzling in her side hair. "Sweet and mellow, sweeter than a flower in May . . . ," Lady hum-

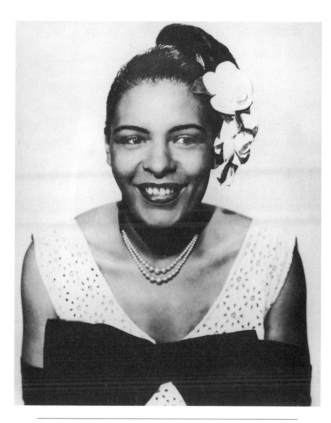

Billie Holiday with her signature gardenia pinned in place.

CORBIS/BETTMAN

sang, moving deeper into the spaces between the notes. Jolted by the smell of burning hair, she pulled the curling iron away, and a big chunk of hair went with it. "Time to go on," a man shouted through the door. "A flower in May" still resonating through her mind, Lady sent Sims to fetch a large bloom from the Three Deuces down the street. Back then, nightclub check-room girls sold flowers. Sims came back with a gardenia, Billie pinned it in her hair, and a star's signature style was born.

FAIR PLAY

As beauty culturists were developing dekinking formulas to tame the hair, others were experimenting with concoctions to lighten dark skin. In her 1919 pamphlet, *A Complete Course in Hair Straightening and Beauty Culture,* Mrs. B. S. Lync of Memphis, Tennessee, offers three face-bleaching formulas.

■ **Face Bleach No. 1**

Hydrogen peroxide 4 oz., citric acid solution 1 dram, almond meal 2 drams, Tr. benzain 8 drops. Mix and apply with the tips of the fingers before retiring at night. In the morning wash the face with warm water.

■ **Face Bleach No. 2**

Bichloride of Mercury 2 grains, sugar of lead 10 grains, water 4 ounces. Mix and apply at night with soft cloth.

■ **Face Bleach No. 3**

Zinc oxide 1/2 dram, sugar of lead 10 grains, Spr. lavender 1 dram, Tr. Benzain 1/2 dram, pure water to make 4 ounces. Mix and apply with soft cloth, night and morning.

IN OTHER WORDS . . .

KITCHEN: The hair on the nape of the neck, which is generally shorter and kinkier than the rest of the hair. As in: "Madam Walker just came over." "Oh yeah, well, she forgot to walk through your kitchen!"

IT ALL COMES DOWN TO THE KITCHEN

Henry Louis Gates Jr.

We always had a gas stove in the kitchen, though electric cooking became fashionable in Piedmont, like using Crest toothpaste rather than Colgate, or watching Huntley and Brinkley rather than Walter Cronkite. But for us it was gas, Colgate, and good ole Walter Cronkite, come what may. We used gas partly out of loyalty to Big Mom, Mama's mama, because she was mostly blind and still loved to cook, and she could feel her way better with gas than with electric.

But the most important thing about our gas-equipped kitchen was that Mama used to do hair there. She had a "hot comb"—a fine-toothed iron instrument with a long wooden handle—and a pair of iron curlers that opened and

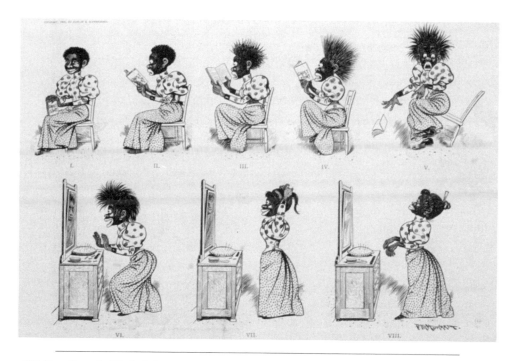

"Taking Out the Kinks." An engraving ca. 1895 by F. M. Howarth Keppler & Schwarzmann demonstrates why black women, with the development of hair-straightening processes, began to distance themselves from stereotypical imagery of black hair and features.

CORBIS

closed like scissors: Mama would put them into the gas fire until they glowed. You could smell those prongs heating up.

I liked what that smell meant for the shape of my day. There was an intimate warmth in the women's tones as they talked with my mama while she did their hair. I knew what the women had been through to get their hair ready to be "done," because I would watch Mama do it to herself. How that scorched kink could be transformed through grease and fire into a magnificent head of wavy hair was a miracle to me. Still is.

Mama would wash her hair over the sink, a towel wrapped 'round her shoulders, wearing just her half-slip and her white bra. (We had no shower until we moved down Rat Tail Road into Doc Wolverton's house, in 1954.) After she had dried it, she would grease her scalp thoroughly with blue Bergamot hair grease, which came in a short, fat jar with a picture of a beautiful colored lady on it. It's important to grease your scalp real good, my mama would explain, to keep from burning yourself.

Of course, her hair would return to its natural kink almost as soon as the hot water and shampoo hit it. To me, it was another miracle how hair so "straight" would so quickly become kinky again once it even approached some water.

My mama had only a few "clients" whose heads she "did"—and did, I think, because she enjoyed it, rather than for the few dollars it brought in. They would sit on one of our red plastic kitchen chairs, the kind with the shiny metal legs, and brace themselves for the process. Mama would stroke that red-hot iron, which by this time had been in the gas fire for half an hour or more, slowly but firmly through their hair, from scalp to strand's end. It made a scorching, crinkly sound, leaving in its wake the straightest of hair strands, each of them standing up long and tall but drooping at the end, like the top of a heavy willow tree. Slowly, steadily, with deftness and grace, Mama's hands would transform a round mound of Odetta kink into a darkened swamp of everglades. The Bergamot made the hair shiny; the heat of the hot iron gave it a brownish red cast. Once all the hair was as straight as God allows kink to get, Mama would take the well-heated curling iron and twirl the straightened strands into more or less loosely wrapped curls. She claimed that she owed her strength and skill as a hairdresser to her wrists, and her little finger would poke out the way it did when she sipped tea. Mama was a southpaw, who wrote upside down and backward to produce the cleanest, roundest letters you've ever seen.

The "kitchen" she would all but remove from sight with a pair of shears bought for this purpose. Now the *kitchen* was the room in which we were sitting, the room where Mama did hair and washed clothes, and where each of us bathed in a galvanized tub. But the word has another meaning, and the "kitchen" I'm speaking of now is the very kinky bit of hair at the back of the head, where the neck meets the shirt collar. If there ever was one part of our African past that resisted assimilation, it was the kitchen. No matter how hot the iron, no matter how powerful the chemical, no matter how stringent the mashed-potatoes-and-lye formula of a man's "process," neither God nor woman nor Sammy Davis Jr. could straighten the kitchen. The kitchen was permanent, irredeemable, invincible kink. Unassimilably African. No matter what you did, no matter how hard you tried, nothing could dekink a person's kitchen. So you trimmed it off as best you could.

When hair had begun to "turn," as they'd say, or return to its natural kinky glory, it was the kitchen that turned first. When the kitchen started creeping up the back of the neck, it was time to get your hair done again. The kitchen around the back, and nappy edges at the temples . . .

My mother furtively examined my daughters' kitchens whenever we went home for a visit in the early eighties. It became a game between us. I had told her not to do it, because I didn't like the politics it suggested of "good" and "bad" hair. "Good" hair was straight. "Bad" hair was kinky. Even in the late sixties, at the height of Black Power, most people could not bring themselves to say "bad" for "good" and "good" for "bad." They still said that hair like white hair was "good," even if they encapsulated it in a disclaimer like "what we used to call 'good.'"

So Maggie would be seated in her high chair, throwing food this way and that, and Mama would be cooing about how cute it all was, remembering how I used to do the same thing, and wondering whether Maggie's flinging her food with her left hand meant that she was going to be a southpaw too. When my daughter was just about covered with Franco-American Spaghetti-Os, Mama would seize the opportunity and wipe her clean, dipping her head, tilted to one side, down under the back of Maggie's neck. Sometimes, if she could get away with it, Mama'd even rub a curl between her fingers, just to make sure that her bifocals had not deceived her. Then she'd sigh with satisfaction and relief, thankful that her prayers had been answered. No kink . . . yet.

THE KINK THAT WINKED
Cynthia Colbert

> *A story of how
> a simple trip to
> the ladies room,
> to primp, powder
> and perfume*

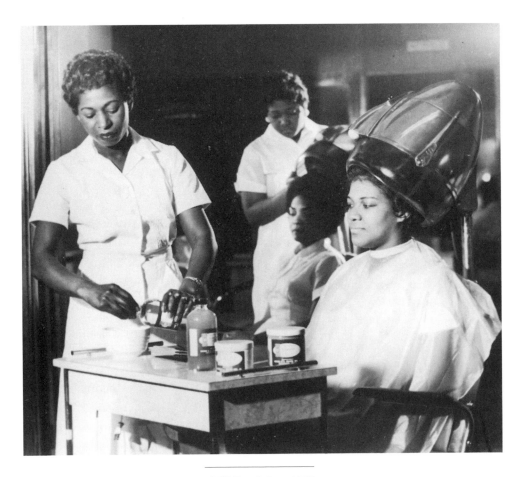

A Walker Salon, 1950s.

MADAM C. J. WALKER COLLECTION/INDIANA HISTORICAL SOCIETY

(givin' it my all)
almost turned into a brawl.
There
it sat
that
one nappy
hap-hap-happy
nap—
like it's sayin'
look at me
I think it may
have even winked
that kink
beside the sink.
Then suddenly—
blond squeals
reel and peel
rollin'
over
over
and over
the stalls
"EEE-YEW
LOOK
A PUBIC HAIR—"

!!??!!!

Oh—no—they—didn't . . .

i blinked
teeterin'

on the brink

and again

i swear the kink winked

now i'm changin' the venue

of this here menu

pondered the fine

saw the headline

pictures of me

after the crime

a number rests

on my chest

me facin' west

LOCAL WRITER

QUITE A FIGHTER

moved to the bowl

eyes

hips

roll

like jelly

ready to jam

bam

move over—ma'am

well no time like the present

me so pleasant

and they like peasants

put in their places

stupid looks on their faces

as i began to comb

my nappy

hap-hap-happy

naps

one fell

two fell

then three
beside the sink
and i think
they may have
even winked.

CAN'TCHA-DON'TCHA HAIR:
Can'tcha comb it; Don'tcha try.

TENDERHEADED: A condition in which the scalp is very sensitive to the combing, tugging, and pulling of the hair. Tears often accompany it.

HOT PROPERTY

Miss Corine's Shop was situated in a small storefront, in between Pitts Funeral Home and Fat Daddy's Rib Shack. . . . On top of looking good, Miss Corine could put a hot curl in the shortest, nappiest of naps and untangle thick, sassy hair on a tenderheaded chile without a single tear. Some called her a miracle worker.

—Shay Youngblood, *Big Mama Stories*

• 2000 •

Ethnic hair-care products (purchased by consumers) reaches $534 million, while personal care services for black women—primarily money spent at hair salons—hits $1.4 billion.

—*Target Market News*

SURPRISE, SURPRISE

This presumption of light skin / "good hair" also accounted for the time a new beautician rinsed the soap out of my locks to discover a thickly tangled brown mass instead of the limply obedient curls she'd expected. "She's too light to be growing some shit like this," she hissed to her friend behind the next chair, rolling her eyes in my direction as if I had willed my roots to crinkle just to fuck with her Friday.

—from *Hairpeace*, Pearl Cleage

TENDERHEADED,
or Rejecting the Legacy of Being Able to Take It
Meg Henson Scales

THE QUESTION—

You Tenderheaded?
reaches from blackberry depths
to millennia of recalcitrant beadabees.
It is the nomenclature of
dark feminine introductions,
that question before the hair
fixing rituals commence,
before the immolation and the ambush,
this naming of things,
"Are you Tenderheaded?"

It's an intimate question, asked impersonally, in either of the traditional standing or sitting poses. When she sits, set there between her legs, your limbs mix and slop, dripping down the sides of beds and davenports, arms over legs, which clasp in an accidental embrace of loving abstract Africania, marvelous.

When she stands, your head nestles against the soft pooch of her abdomen as she becomes totally hands and arms, completely for your "Tenderhead—or Not"? The musk can be scandalous from here, intertwined, it enslaves you in that chair, even the memory of it.

"Are you Tenderheaded?"

Hanging in your answer, the neck can easily become a fulcrum and the hair a lever, absently directing the face, unnaturally, perpendicular to the spine, providing tension against one's self. Enduring this is total macha, and it only occurs when one answers that all-important question in the negative: "No, I'm Not Tenderheaded," the unsaid being: I can take it.

This denial of sensation in the head and neck, this disallowing one's physical pain or discomfort solely for the convenience of one's "stylist," is a most disingenuous and underexamined cultural construct. In girlhood, it readies the child for the merciless role of the much-vaunted yet antihero strongblackwoman;

under whose guise, a blank emotional palate is assumed, probably for the first time.

Strongblackwoman's most striking characteristics are her gross displays of endurance and the absence of a personal agenda. The strongblackwoman lives for (and sometimes through) others, and is culturally valued in direct proportion to her personal sacrifice. Strongblackwomen are the astronauts, the most right stuff of American martyrdom.

If we then consider Tenderheadedness as a paradigm for self-worth in black girlhood, we can perhaps understand something more of what makes American black women so specifically disparaged from within and without.

There is no tenderness in this march to the bottom of the hierarchy, just as there are no tangible rewards in pursuing an elusive "hair fixing" based upon European aesthetics. Not being Tenderheaded is a pain preparation, not an analgesic. Its supposition of crime (felony napistry) and punishment (corrective straightening) is curious enough, without its extorted confession of neuropathy ("No, I am not Tenderheaded").

Most American women suffer for beauty/acceptance, though none as trumpeted as this monstrous strongblackwoman fetish, that wrestles with us, within and without, exacting. Even the most-told martyr of American womantales, the Jewishmother, does not get her hair pulled and burned in the course of her daily toilette, and she typically would not countenance such an imposition.

If we examine the cartoonish cinematic depictions of the sultry temptress/crack ho, or the media's societally dependent breeder, we find no one intrinsically good in the storehouse of accepted black women's repertoire, until we find Mammy. Needless to say, Mammy is never Tenderheaded.

The raison d'être of the strongblackwoman was never to be inconsequential, or to live a life unburdened with self-interest; it was a survival tactic, utilized under the most trying circumstances in contemporary history.

Now strongblackwoman is an expectation, it is the math of the myth of our horribleness. It is not surprising, then, that any strongblackwoman worth her high blood pressure and obesity feels that any time spent on herself is time wasted.

Following the gangsta beat, African-American youth culture has been in rapt accord about the utter dispensability of its female members, with its bitch/ho

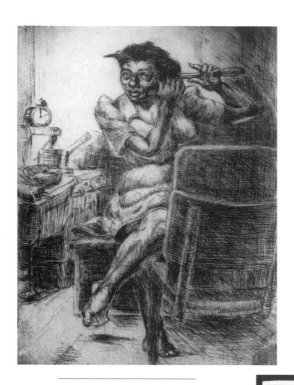

*Saturday Night, an etching
by Dox Thrash, ca. 1940.*

MARY'S ● BEAUTY ● SHOPPE

HOURS

8:30 TO 9:00 CLOSED TUESDAYS AT 6:00

STANDARED PRICE LIST

SHAMPOO & PRESS	.50
SHAMPOO PRESS & CURLS	65&.75
SHAMPOO PRESS & WAVE	1.00&1.25
COMB PRESS & WAVE	.75
HARD " & "	1.00
MARCEL WAVE	.50&.75
FINGER "	.50
CROQUINOLE WAVE	.50&.75
SHAMPOO PRESS & CROQUINOLE	1.00&1.25
PLAIN SCALP TREATMET	.15
DANDRUF " "	.25
END CURLS	.25
MANICURE	.25
HAND & ARM MASSAGE	.25
" & " BLEACH	.35
FACIAL PLAIN	.50
" PACK	.75
EYE BROW ACH	.25
ARCH FREE WITH FACAIL	

IT PAYS ● TO LOOK
● YOUR BEST ●

A price list from Mary's Beauty Shoppe.

nomenclature and corporate backing. In that hostile terrain, it is comprehensible why so many young women cloak themselves in weight and children; and why so many defend the vile forms that denigrate them, under the witless guise of "telling it like it is."

What we know about youth, their individual possibilities, and our collective past, makes not being Tenderheaded a very poignant lie, especially for our girls. Strongblackwomen have not been getting fat on their pain and hardship, they have been starving on it. We should tell them these things.

The Tenderheads, in contrast, perceive themselves in an adoring, a more giving light, and they reflect this, with more repose than bearing, more portrait than posture. They expertly define how little distress one should be willing to endure for the sake of appearances, with a hugged knee or slightly shrunken shoulder, their untwisted necks all soft and pliant.

They are absolutely no help whatsoever to the napaloosa tasks at hand, which is anathema to strongblackwomen who unnaturally are, of course, all the help. The Tenderheaded offerings are meager, yet each is gold, for they are Tenderheaded, and that must be acknowledged.

The needed play of ballast and weights, when extruding the naps from their natural state, doesn't even concern the Tenderhead—under the best of circumstances, their hair retains a hint of bushy nostalgia, a pleasurable contradiction to the parallelogram order being forced upon such anarchic tangle—and still they are complimented on their mundane hair achievements, still!

The Tenderheaded's lips are dahlias, complaints and sighs pouring from their fluted depths, for she knows from practice that complaint is the cornerstone of relief, especially in this mise-en-scène of napistry.

Each sigh that drafts from her effulgent lips should be seized upon and attended to, because the Tenderhead is likely to just up and leave altogether, before the scalp is greased, before the doobee is pinned, the hair tracked or burned or yanked or washed and blown, she might just hat up and go.

Harriet Tubman was Tenderheaded.

There are also stories of the cruelties visited upon some hapless Tenderheads, but we simply won't tell them here, since they can easily be guessed.

During the actual "fixing," their ears flatten against their Tenderheads, drinking in the browned and oval tones of whoever so gently dresses their hair. The Tenderheads are talked through their stylings, whereas the Nots are stalked through theirs. For that betrayal of sensation, the yelp or the ouch! Let a whimper emerge from a Not, and the rebuke is as swift and triumphant as with the swatting of a fly—"I thought you said you weren't Tenderheaded!" is the very closest a Not will get to compassion. Instead, chastened and silenced for another round of scorching or yanking, the naperial cauterization recommences, O Africania!

It can go dominatrix in a heartbeat—you in a kitchen chair, and she standing, imperious, brandishing a plastic comb in striking zone from you, freshly washed and trapped. A stovetop glows near, with heated irons smoking, and you have only yourself to blame.

She might lean herself into you as she works, and she might squint warmly through the halo of smoke your hair has become, but so much lies in the challenge before her, this prelude to the scorching of nappy tendrils, the hyphen of blister to come on the curl of an ear, this delicate kitchen of the neck, exposed . . . Are you Tenderheaded?

There is something about suffering and melanin and estrogen that has been added up incorrectly and then mispronounced. We are not included in white feminist theory, we are not the women of the National Organization of Women, we are the ones ignored in their polls and census, when they say "blacks and women." Our struggles are the most bloodied and extended; and our stories the least honored. Within that context, as long as Not being Tenderheaded masquerades as the greater good, it is being kidnapped out of context and used as a cudgel. It says, if the strongblackwoman is "able to take it," here's some more!

To consider Tenderheadedness with not taking it then, is to potentially disabuse ourselves of the entire strongblackwoman hoodwinking altogether. History positively exhorts us to understand that once any people have had enough, when that word alone can fully describe their collective response to oppression, those same people will either become more proficient at eliminating the sources of their despair or they'll take it to their graves, taking it with them, since people insist upon getting used to just about anything, even genocide.

Rosa Parks, another celebrated Tenderhead, spearheaded a movement based totally upon her unwillingness to be "strong" enough to take it—indeed her strength was in her utter rejection of taking it, the consequences of not taking it mattering less than her personal safety.

When reminded of human sentience, no matter how nappy one's crown is or isn't, from the lushly coarse to the natural wave to the imperial afros, to the beadabee buckshot; everyone is Tenderheaded, or simply, just about everyone has feelings or sensation, even in the head and neck, and particularly in the heart. This person with no declared sensation in her head and shoulders, who is "Not Tenderheaded," is not so subtly investing in the juggernaut of the strongblackwoman, and she is being ignored.

All that power in our collusions, sitting there between each other's legs, dripping down our bedsides and burning in our kitchens, all that juice is being wasted. It would be much better to simply love during those moments.

In my girlhood, I was not Tenderheaded, because I had so-called "good hair" and was not allowed to be "funny" about it. It was also part penance, since I was considered ungrateful for my "good hair" in the first place.

My mother would braid my head in two, quite lovingly, as long as I wasn't freshly washed, which changed my hair from just getting done to getting fixed. But usually, with me between her legs, clasping her knees, facing out, a sotto voce hugging took place, nice, if not wonderful.

She'd sometimes compliment me on my hair as if I'd finally done something right, and I believed in the softness she said it had, that I'd done good, and sometimes she'd scratch my scalp so exquisitely with the tail of the comb, my chest would flame. We did my hair anywhere, but most memorably, wonderfully, in her sewing room in that basement, watching baseball on a black-and-white television.

Summers, my mother wore black Capri pants and a black bra, smoking Tareytons and sipping baby Olympia beers while she sewed. All of her sewing gear was set up in half of the rec room in our basement, so the windows were near the ceilings, which were low, and all the other furniture was parted-out junk from the rest of the house. Being a classic strongblackwoman herself, my mother never met a used piece of shit that wouldn't do better than something nice and/or new for herself.

As her only daughter, I was expected to then graciously receive all of the lovely things she couldn't accept for herself—like the calf-length, fully lined, fire-engine-red wool melton cape she surprised me with in the August of my eighth grade.

To be Tenderheaded under these conditions would have been reprehensible, and even I knew, in the eye of my own adolescent chaos, that the Good Fight lay in claiming myself a Not, so I did. It was a moot declaration for a long time, as our regimen was uncomplicated and predictable, the only variable being bangs, made from a Goody pink foam curler, the kind that snap when they close.

With a little Three Flowers Brilliantine, my bangs would straighten and curl overnight, with only the Goody roller and some water, but because it aroused questions of racial purity from my Negro friends, I kept this shortcut around the straightening comb to myself—no one but my family knew.

Since my father and my twin brother had too many "white features" for these same tribalists, there was a strong perception amongst these same great people that I too was almost certainly racially underendowed, and that my brown skin was just a cover for something paler and sinister.

I was mortified when my bang secret was discovered by one of my classmates in front of the water fountain one afternoon at school. We'd just pulled a particularly rigorous safety patrol in the rain, and I'd thoughtlessly wrung them out in the fountain and curled them under with my fingers.

I straightened up, and we were head to head; I was looking dead into her drenched messy naps, gone (as they used to say), plastered on her forehead as she stared into my fraudulent and tubular bang roll, freshly turned.

Hair perjury was a serious offense, and she didn't believe my lie or my hastily botched bang roll or my compliments on her go-go boots for even a moment, but I'd reached a watershed resolution: I would not be outcast on the grounds of something so ludicrous as "good hair," not if I could help it.

When my mother started pressing my hair, at my insistence, in that loathsome seventh grade, she wept in the kitchen, burning me, my ears, my hair, "Just ruining your beautiful hair!" she cried. Later, she blew Tareyton smoke in my face and told me that since I'd started "frying" my hair, I'd never be able to stop, and I suddenly started noticing things about her, like how fat her behind looked as she walked away from me.

"What'd you do to your hair?" they said at school, and they were pleased; my hair looked terrible, burned and greasy, and we were one, me and my friends; or at least we were "we" again. This pain was perhaps my first taste of being something very similar to a credit to my race, and every bit as unrewarding.

My hair became an ordeal, more strongblackwomanly, thankless, unpleasant, never during a baseball game and for the first time, always near a heat source. If I happened to flinch at the sizzle of an ear, or a scorching of the kitchen under the irons, I was reminded that this was my desire, my transgression—that I could have stuck with the braids and the bangs—and "I thought you said you weren't Tenderheaded!"

There was apparently no turning back, no "passing" after one takes that fateful stand as being Not Tenderheaded. I was doomed. From the hot seat, I started noticing my cousin, who had always been Tenderheaded. We occasionally had our hair done at the same time, since our mothers were sisters, but I was always long gone by the time she was done, since her hair seemed to take forever.

Now that my own hair needed more "fixing," I realized that what had been taking so long was this tremendous ass-kissing she was getting, right in front of God and everyone, her with her Tenderhead. She'd sit between my aunt's legs like a soft golden Buddha, her beautiful long bush in rays extending, or parted like farm land in more manageable sections as the fixing progressed—her in her catbird seat!

"Are you OK?" my aunt would ask solicitously, and my cousin might even say, "No! It hurts!!" and other flabbergasting backtalk. How she'd miraculously be invited to rest even, to stretch her pampered legs! To top it off, she was roundly congratulated for getting her hair done, for being so "good" about it and all, whereas I was simply Not Tenderheaded, for all my hurt.

I protested to my mother about this Not clause hanging (literally) over my head. She agreed in part, saying that I was, in effect, a junior kind of zygote version of the strongblackwoman, and therefore, while my pain was real, it either didn't matter or just confirmed itself by being, Zen-like.

She then implied, without actually calling her one, that my cousin was a slight pain in the ass with that Tenderheaded business, and that's about all there was to it. She also offered that she knew I could take it—I thanked her for that—and that anyway, no daughter of hers would be Tenderheaded anyway, it was genetic or something.

This worked for me until soon after our conversation, I watched my mother do my cousin's hair. "Are you OK?" she asked the golden girl. "How's this, Sweetie?" she petted, she cooed. "You were real good, honey!" she said when she was done, sweat pouring from her from the effort, as my cousin floated out of our basement like a butterfly.

There are more arduous tasks before us than to be tender to each other, especially when we're there between each other, enveloped, doing our heads. In all likelihood, there is no greater climate possible for the devastating teachings of strongblackwomanhood than the ones given in those accidental embraces.

If we remember that this overabundance of misery and usury and taking it are how we got this way, then we can intuit, if not see from here, that there is no freedom in that bag, that there never was, and we can renounce it altogether.

How profoundly we must delve, even to find the smallest bit of tenderness for ourselves! Unfolding these dormant capacities for gentleness and compassion for ourselves will certainly engage new mechanisms in our living that aren't so concerned with suffering in the first place.

When we bury the mythological strongblackwoman expectation, even one inhumanity at a time, it can still rescue us from the massive belittlements we suffer daily; each time, changing the math, adding us up. It is self-evident that we must now, for all of us, become Tenderheaded. Yes.

Baby Hair

We are born blissfully ignorant of concepts like good hair and bad, kinks and curls. But in a few years' time, without anyone to teach us, as they do with numbers and nursery rhymes, we learn from the clues. A passing comment, a sideways glance, communicate belonging, exclusion, beauty, invisibility. As we whisper into the ears of future generations, what will we say?

BABY HAIR
Constance Nichols

*I took a peek for the very first time
At the tiny brown mite on the bed.
He blinked his eyes and doubled plump fists,
and I ran to his mother and said,
"The most cunning baby I ever did see,"
But she, lying patiently there,
Touched my arm and with anxious voice
Whispered, "Does he have good hair?"*

A DAY AT THE BEACH
Kay Brown

During summers, when I was a girl, my aunt used to take me with her to spend a few weeks in Glen Cove, Long Island. She had a friend there who owned a house that was walking distance from the beach. One day in the early 1940s, when I was about nine, I was sitting on the sand, toasting in the sun and

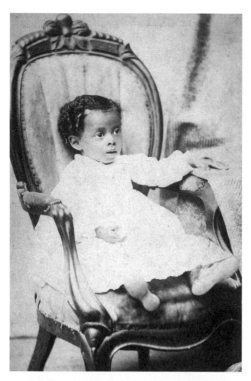

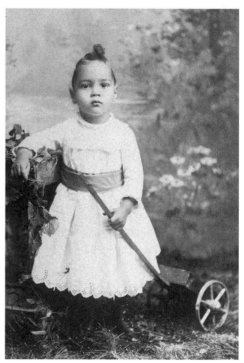

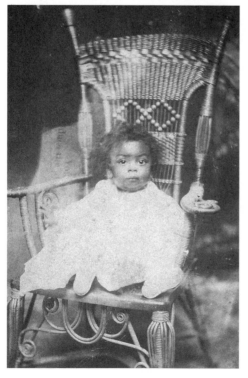

Nineteenth-century tots.

DERRICK BEARD COLLECTION

watching the incoming waves. Glen Cove seemed a long way from New York City, where I lived, and I was happy to be away from the crowds and the noise.

"Don't forget your bathing cap," my aunt reminded me, as I rose from the blanket and headed toward the water. "Your mother just did your hair."

Like I needed reminding? Just before we'd left, my mother had pressed and curled my hair, burning the tips of both ears this time, even though she was a professional beautician.

Pouting, I doubled back for the bathing cap and pulled it down on my head. Slowly, I waded into the water. I didn't really know how to swim, so I tried different strokes, hoping to teach myself. Of course my head went underwater. Suddenly, I felt it seeping into the bathing cap. Oh, my God! I panicked. What had I done? There had to be a hole in the cap or something.

I stood in the water, wondering what to do, my toes pushing into the soft surface below my feet. Then, on a whim I could never explain, I pulled off the bathing cap and ducked my entire head into the water. Shoot, I had blown it anyway. For the rest of the day, I had a great time, splashing, trying to float as the waves wriggled through my curls, and feeling as free as the birds sailing above me.

• 1900s •

In Buckingham County, Virginia, a black woman was visited by a neighbor who was blind. The blind woman settled down by the hearth and reached out to greet her neighbor's daughter who had string-wrapped hair. Feeling the girl's head, the blind woman said, "You musta wrapped this child's head real tight because her eyes are standing on her forehead!"

The pickaninny Topsy is born as Harriet Beecher Stowe's novel *Uncle Tom's Cabin; or, Life among the Lowly* is published. Stowe writes that when Topsy arrived at her new master's household, her "woolly hair was braided in sundry little tails, which stuck out in every direction." The child was dispatched to the mammy of the household, who forthwith clipped her hair. "Shorn of all the little braided tails wherein her heart had delighted," Topsy was deprived of an element of her antic charm.

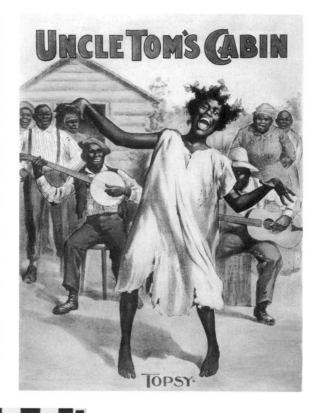

Life among the Lowly.

THE GRANGER COLLECTION

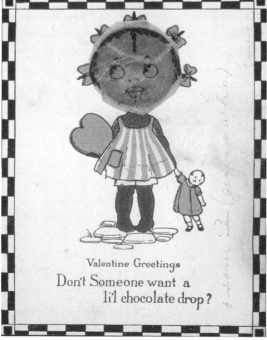

Valentine Greetings
Don't Someone want a
li'l chocolate drop?

DERRICK BEARD COLLECTION

LEARNING THE LANGUAGE OF MY DAUGHTER'S HAIR
Peter Harris

In 1987 I learned to love braiding my daughter's hair. That's the year that Adenike, then seven years old, stepped off the plane to begin a summer visit with me in California. She was holding Jessica, the teddy bear she'd brought for protection and comfort, and wearing two neat plaits on either side of her head. Within a week's time, her hair needed washing. The task seemed simple enough. But when I untwined her plaits, my girl looked like Chaka Khan after three encores. Scared me to death.

I had to tame all that? Wash it, dress it, part it, plait it? It was summertime, but the living was not easy. It quickly dawned on me that I had never braided hair in my life. Now, growing up in D.C. I had seen little sisters plaiting each other's hair, or watched as young women in high school sat between each other's legs and spun three strands into gold. A lot of my buddies during the seventies had girlfriends braid their hair before basketball games, or just so they could style. Once I even had my own hair cornrowed before a high school baseball game so my cap could sit firmly on my otherwise flyaway 'fro. And the spring before Ade arrived, I had practiced by weaving, unraveling, and reweaving yarn hanging from a bedpost. But neither memories nor macramé could prepare me for my baby's briar patch. Her mother's words rang in my ears: "She's very very tenderheaded!"

That first session took more than an ouch-filled hour. Throughout the next week, she cried a lot as I tortured her with my dreaded comb and brush. Mornings were especially tense. Tightening up her hair became the A.M. demand that fixing breakfast and lunch could never be. I even stopped playing the radio or listening to Earth, Wind & Fire records, although music had fueled my morning ritual for years.

In the days ahead, as I made the rounds to introduce Ade to friends, at least one of my sister-girls rolled her eyes at my daughter's hair.

"Why don't you bring her on over to my house," she gently suggested.

I told her no out of pride and continued to hack away.

I learned my first lesson about handling hair from my partner's eighteen-year-old daughter during a weekend visit to their home. Before a Saturday outing, she unbraided what I just knew had been a hip ponytail. She combed through kinks in Ade's head that I never knew existed. The reworked do was obviously better than the one I had created. I slumped, but my friend explained without sneering that I hadn't been combing all the way to the roots. She advised me to comb through small sections at a time—starting with the ends—to limit the pressure on the scalp.

Made sense.

I thought I had the hang of it. But later that week, somebody at day camp unhooked Ade's plaits and substituted two smart cornrows.

I got to soul-searching again. Why didn't I let somebody cornrow me out my constriction and be done with it? I was feeling out my league, locked out of the circle of wisdom where all the grooming secrets are passed on. Deep down, I was also plain embarrassed: There I was, a grown man, and I couldn't even fix my own daughter's hair.

Once I moved past shame, then I arrived at pissed! Here I was braiding Ade's hair, and women were redoing my styles without asking my permission, or even if I wanted their help. Turn the tables. Let me or some other man—day-care director, boyfriend, husband, or candy man on the corner—put his hands on one of their daughters, and be talking about, "Girl, I'm just doing a touch-up"! Sister be cussing him out, dialing 911, and feeling around for a knife—all the while holding her daughter close, redoing the hairstyle, and wiping imaginary sleep out the child's eyes!

As mad as this double standard made me, I have to admit, doing hair was proving too tough for the kid. Then I had a breakthrough. It came after an intense conversation with another woman friend, who encouraged me to keep trying. Despite the tears, my friend assured me, Adenike appreciated my hard work and would remember my determination all her life. Then, fingering her own magnificent dreads, she fondly reminisced about the snap, crackle, and pop of *her* mother's hands.

That night I dreamed that I had been going about it all wrong: I saw braiding as a chore, instead of as an opportunity for special intimacy with my daughter. I was too tentative. Every time she whimpered, I eased up and brushed only the surface of her hair.

My dream also offered me some practical advice:

Use more Dax Jack! Don't make her Little Richard or nobody, but spread a little more sheen, boy! Soften the hair so the girl won't need a Mister Ray hair weave after you comb to the roots.

I had a New Attitude at our next session. We had gone swimming, and I got down, if I do say so myself.

After I used shampoo and conditioner, her hair draped damply, defiantly. But this time, with comb in hand, I took a deep breath and easily separated small portions until her scalp peeked out. Section by section, I parted her hair, fingering dressing down each row, until her crown had a fragrant glow to it. Handling Ade's hair gave me chills. Slowly I braided, and to my satisfaction—my sasafaction, to borrow from soul crooner Clarence Carter—deepened twist by tug by criss by cross. I transformed her hair into patterned plaits. Through four well-woven braids, she didn't moan at all. She looked into the mirror, rubbed her hands over the job, and nodded approvingly.

I was fired up. Once again, I felt under control as a father. A part of me—quiet as it's kept—was gleeful that black women aren't born knowing how to braid hair. Mostly, though, I felt good reconfirming that with perseverance, dedication and imagination I could learn to speak a loving, painless language to my daughter through her thick, healthy hair.

After that, I even got halfway creative. One hairstyle included a braided ponytail and two other braids hanging from the side that had my baby remarking in an airy, awed little voice: "You can't even see the ponytail unless you hold it up."

I could braid hair. Damn! I felt like I had cracked a code or something. In a way I had: the summer of '87 was a turning point for me and Ade. I mean, it was her first visit with me since me and her mother divorced in 1984. I had expected her in the summers of '85 and '86, but custody battles shoved those visits to the back burner. Before Adenike finally came, the only real time I'd had with her was in her first year and a half of life. Even then, I was working out of town, away from our Baltimore home.

By the time Ade visited in '87, she didn't really remember those days. She only knew me through pictures and gifts through the mail, or the occasional long-distance calls in which I talked and she listened, or she spoke with curious detachment in her little-girl voice. Those calls only left me hollow.

I missed her, though, because I remembered what she couldn't. Feeding her.

Changing her diaper. Pushing her stroller in the neighborhood around our East Baltimore row house. Letting her fall asleep on my chest. Catnapping myself on our queen-size bed, while she crawled across my face or sat beside me, playing with a toy.

I used to give her baths. Even took baths with her, along with the miniature boat, yellow rubber duck, and plastic soap dish. Man, those baths were peaceful communions. Time slowed to a caring pace. I remember every detail. I'd run the water—warm, but leaning toward cool—until it was high enough only to reach her chest when she sat down.

Once, when she was sixteen months, I remember hollering her nickname down the hall while the water ran: "Ahhhdaaaaayyyy." She waddles out from the bedroom to meet my voice. She sees my toothbrush sticking from my mouth. Her eyes light up, 'cause she's been "brushing" her four front teeth. Pointing toward my mouth, Adenike babbles a request for her brush, which is an orange miniature of my white one. I grab her hand, and we walk to the bathroom. I turn off the water, then hand her the brush full of paste. With her attention diverted, I plop her into the water so she's sitting, even though she always prefers to stand. The toothbrush sticks from her mouth like a toothpick.

Squirming, grabbing the side of the tub, she pulls herself up anyway. With her right hand clutching the rim of the tub, she gathers her balance and stands in triumph. Facing me, she's my grinning Pot Belly Baby. Her pudgy brown left hand holds the brush. Almost falling, her mouth becomes a soft oval of surprise. I can see her gapped top two teeth and her bottom two looking like erect white sentinels. She regains her balance and her black black eyes, with even blacker pupils, dance in some private merry triumph. I crack up at my naked baby clown.

Memories like these fueled me, soothed me, sustained me, when I moved out of our Baltimore house and eventually to California. If Ade remembered anything of baths and naps with Daddy, she didn't show it by the time she visited me in June 1987. Often, "Mommy" slipped out her mouth before she asked me questions. And the first time she fell—while she skipped ahead of me across an empty street—she wailed such a pitiful "Mommy" that I damn near wished her mother would materialize myself and help me check her scraped hands and knees.

Since she was only going to spend two months of that summer with me, I desperately wanted to communicate and commune with her in a special and particular way, so we could lock our thing in the pocket. I wanted to be her daddy, not just her father, complete with our own rituals/language/intimacy, the way I was with her brother, who had been living with me since the divorce.

Looking back on that summer, it's no question that learning the secret language of braiding her hair allowed me and Ade to become daddy and daughter. It was the mutual beginning of our most precious memories. Time began for us after braiding.

Since 1987, we have had miles but no distance between us. We have developed a new confidence, an understanding of how we can, and will, work together to stay close and really get to know each other. We've learned each other's moods and body language. We've developed our own style of discipline and celebration.

During our subsequent visits, I could sense when she really wanted to sleep with me—because missing Mommy, or the group of girlfriends she'd left behind, hung on her too heavy to handle. Or she definitely understood that when I said I hated whining, I hated whining! And that if she really wanted something, she'd best speak up directly and confidently, 'cause if she whined for it I turned deaf, dumb and blind.

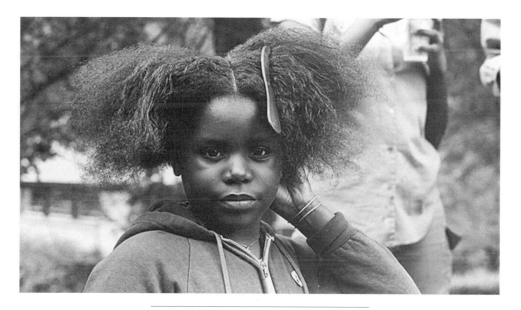

Comb as accessory, 1970s Brooklyn, New York.

OWEN FRANKEN/CORBIS

She and I learned how to hang. I cooked and cleaned, read to her, took her shopping, to the movies, said yes, said no, laughed at her jokes, told her punch lines of my own, got great big hugs, heard bits of gossip from mom's household, held her hand when we hit the street, bought her En Vogue and Bobby Brown tapes, and played, as I did for all my kids and any youngster within earshot of my turntable, all my classic Temptations records.

In the summer of '90 I took Ade, then ten, and her then-thirteen-year-old brother Ketema to Florida. During our chlorine-and-salt-water-soaked vacation, I braided her hair every day. By then, me and Ade were duet partners. She'd ask for a style, I'd do it. If we were in a hurry to get out the house to go, say, to Disney World, I'd whip her hair into a style that wouldn't come loose with all the running and sweating and waiting in lines. If she'd just washed her hair after we'd all had a dip in the pool in the muggy Florida night, we'd take our time and watch a movie on HBO, the rhythm of combing through hair matching the sundown ease between mellow partners sure of their confidence in each other.

In the summer of '93, Ade turned thirteen. Of course, by then she wanted to style her own hair (even into styles that required hot curlers, which I couldn't get to with my natural- and dreadlock-loving ass). But I couldn't help but dig her independence and creativity. Besides, I was confident (please God!) that all those braiding sessions, the many times I'd taken her to sisters for full-blown cornrows, and the overall, affirmative black vibe of my household would bloom into some consistent natural hairstyle she'd choose for long-term pleasure and reflection.

Meantime, get this, I found myself teasingly spot-checking to make sure she was combing down to the roots. Ain't that a trip! She didn't pay me no mind, either, 'cause she was a big girl. Young woman. Eighth grader. As far from being that caramel toddler in the Baltimore bathtub as I was from being that nervous, second-time father worried that she'd slip out my loving hands and drown in two feet of water.

But I laughed and told her, "You know I can still braid it if I got to," and she cracked up 'cause she knew it was true. She knew her daddy could do her hair. If he wanted to. If she wanted him to!

Looking back, my dreadlocked "counselor" was as right as rain about one thing: braiding Adenike's hair gave me the powerfully intimate way to help my daughter gain confidence in me. These days, I may be out of the hairstyling/hairdressing loop, but in my prime I could ask her to get the comb, brush, and barrettes, and her smile wouldn't hibernate. Sometimes, 'cause turnabout is fair play, and she and I had found what we were looking for, she even sat me down to brush and comb my hair and beard.

At this writing, my daughter, who is now a young woman, wears her hair short. As a member of her college track team (my baby entered the school on a combination academic and athletic scholarship!), she finds it much hipper to sport the wash-and-wear look. Over the years, Adenike has evolved into a powerful, beautiful person, with a sense of humor that delights me. She's also serious and hardworking, and her sensitivity inspires me.

I haven't braided Adenike's hair in years now. Still, I savor the intimacy we created during those times when she squirmed under my hair-hacking, hair-braiding hands. We remain daddy and daddy's baby, you know, having gone beyond just father and daughter, which could have been our fate given the divorce and geographical distance. When we talk by phone or during our visits, we have no taboo subjects. We've grappled with the history of me and her moms, her evolving explorations of sex and relationships, my 40-something life as a single man, her worries, my worries. And of course, we riff on school and sports in that overall silly groove we fall into when we take the time to hang.

HAIR (R)EVOLUTION
Cynthia Colbert

I was eight and every two weeks took the bus
to miss jerrie pearl who "did" hair
in her basement.
smell of burnt hair and grease.
girl, your hair sure is nappy and dirty this time.
what have you been into?

• 1924 •

BANKING ON BABY

Amid a bevy of beauty contests in the 1920s, including the Bobbed Hair Contest sponsored by the Brotherhood of Sleeping Car Porters, the NAACP's W. E. B. Du Bois features the winners of dozens of baby contests on the pages of the *Crisis* magazine. Babies, it turns out, are a real moneymaker. In 1924, for example, NAACP branches in fifteen states raise $9,409. And a year later, seventy-eight such contests yield some $20,000.

—Shane White and Graham White, *Stylin': African American Expressive Culture*

running around with fuzz and naps.
what would folks think?
why, they would think I was just a kid
having all the fun I could get my hands on.
although it would have been nice to have hair
like my friend dixie who sat next to me at school.
hers was all nice and shiny and long and blond.

I was fourteen and wore my psychedelic lime green bell-bottoms
like a badge of honor, but—
something was missing.
I pleaded;
mama, pleeeeeeese
let me wear an afro.
girl why anyone would want to wear that mess,
i'll never know.
running around looking all wild.
what would folks think?
why, they would think I was black, beautiful and
proud, like my girl nikki g.
talkin' about men in their tight, tight pants
and big afros.
and maybe, just maybe, they would know
that I was about black power,
on the order of eldridge and stokely
or huey.
when mama finally said ok,
honey, I had me an afro
that would have made angela davis proud.
painstakingly braided every night.
picked, shaped and patted.

I was sixteen and revlon was calling my name.
had to get a "perm."
and farrah fawcett blond streaks.
then, later, aretha reddish brown.
while others tried alcohol and weed,
I experimented with my hair.
why would you want to perm your hair?
you just want to be like the white girls.
I heard jerilyn barnes' hair fell out
in patches because of that stuff.
no boy wants a bald-headed girl.
what would they think?
maybe they would think I was beautiful
with my shiny, silky hair
parted down the middle and feathered to the back.
with just a few blond streaks around my face.
or maybe they would show me some r–e–s–p–e–c–t
if it was aretha-red.
maybe they wouldn't notice how big my butt
was getting or the breakouts on my face.
i'm just trying to find "me."

I was twenty,
bound by the box that had promised
shiny, silky, even sexy hair.
burning my scalp, my ears, my hair;
a delicious agony
to hair that's mine—and his.
isn't it time to do something to your hair?
getting a little nappy around the edges.
want my wife to look good when we go out.
what would people think?

why, they would think that I was a young housewife
and mother, loving and nurturing,
whose kids and her man are well cared for.
I may be your wife, but these edges are mine.
trust me, I know when my hair needs to be done.
functional when it needs to be
sleek and sexy when I need it to be
I can cook up the bacon,
fry it up in the pan,
and never, never let you forget—
well, you know the rest.

there goes thirty, now here comes forty
enduring this, this what?
one and a half hour ordeal at least twice
a week—shampoo, blow dry, curling iron.
don't they know that a single working mom
wants hair that looks good but is easy to take care of?
fashion with ease.
I'm not that hard to please.
wash and wear hair.
but do I dare?
you work in an office.
a nice relaxed bob is the corporate look.
and it's fairly easy to care for.
if you wore those braids, locks, afro (select one)
to work, why, what would they think?
"they" would probably find it fascinating
as they all seem to think our hair is.
can I touch it?
it doesn't look like it would be so soft.
how do you do that?

▪ 1940 ▪

In his report *Children of Bondage,* Allison Davis details the obsessive hair and color preoccupations of African Americans in New Orleans and Natchez: "Parents and grandparents were extremely concerned about the color and hair-form of the baby, consoling each other if the child were darker or had 'worse' hair than had been expected, and felicitating each other if it was lighter or had 'better' hair than had been expected. Even before the birth of a child, some upper-class and upper-middle-class parents surveyed in minute detail all the possibilities with regard to the child's color and hair-form by recalling these traits in each of their parents and grandparents."

you can do so much with your hair.

and the stares and questions would end

once the novelty wore off.

what would they think?

WHO CARES?

THINGS MY MOTHER NEVER TAUGHT ME
Jacquelyn Long

As I waited impatiently for the adoption of the child I had dreamed of for many years to come through, I studied every aspect of child rearing with an enthusiasm that I should have had when I was a Ph.D. student. It was only after my beautiful five-month-old baby was placed in my arms that I realized the truth of

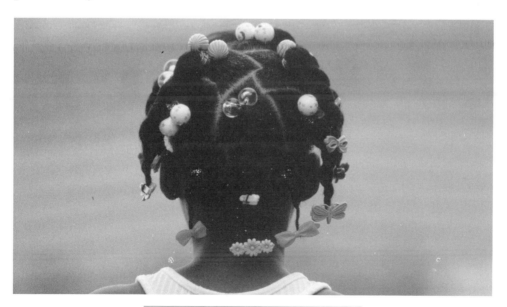

A colorful and pervasive type of African-American folk art.

NATHAN BENN/CORBIS

that old saying about experience being the best teacher. After a few months of searching all my books to determine the significance of Jessica's latest sneeze or rash, I noticed that I could just look at my baby and know when she was out of sorts even when others were assuring me she was fine.

However, as Jessica's hair progressed from baby fine to tightly coiled, I didn't know what to do with it. That I should have also prepared to care for her hair had never occurred to me. And I suppose even if I had thought about it, it would not have made the "Top 100 Things I Need to Know to Be a Good Mom" list. But hair care has turned out to be very important; especially now that Jessica, at age ten, has begun forming her own concept of beauty.

I was born with hair very different from Jessica's. When I was a child, I loved sitting with my mother on the old wooden steps of our house in Lawrenceville, Virginia, getting my hair combed after she'd washed it. Brushing a section around her finger, she made Shirley Temple curls to dry as I played in the sun. Then she'd braid it into two plaits. Once a child who was visiting a neighbor asked me if I pressed my hair. I had no idea what she meant. I had never heard people talk about pressing hair before. A funny expression flickered across her face, and she never answered when I asked her what she meant. Looking back on the incident now, I believe she was confused because she recognized little brown me as being like her—a "Negro" girl—and yet she was just beginning to realize that some black people were born with straight hair.

A lot of people seemed to like my hair. I thought maybe it was because it was longer than that of anyone else I knew—except my mother. Mom's hair fell to the middle of her back. I loved those times when my mother let me wear my hair "out," instead of braided. I felt so special with loose swirling hair that I kept going back to her to get the curl the way it was before I began to play. My parents, concerned about how my behavior might appear to others, began telling me not to talk so much about my hair around other people. This confused me and made me wonder whether there was something wrong with my hair.

When I was a teenager, I was never allowed to participate in hair talk. My friends would complain about the problems they had with their hair. When I tried to mention the terrible times I had with mine, though, they'd laugh and brush me aside. What I was trying to tell them was that I had to spend hours on my hair each time I washed and dried it, and that I spent an hour each night rolling it up, only to have everything ruined if a single roller came out while I

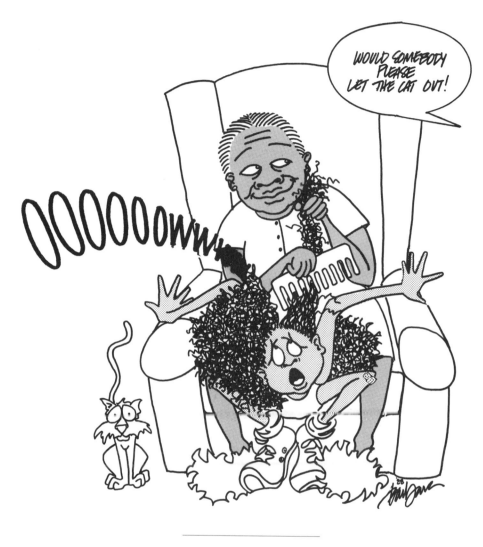

BARBARA BRANDON

slept. I used these extra-bouffant plastic rollers that made my head look twice its normal size.

At Fisk University, I was still banned from the hair-wailing sessions in the dorm because most girls thought I had it too "good." Students told me about the curl in my hair hanging down my back and how it bounced as I walked. I must admit I was flattered. But once, during a semester break when I was stuck on campus with nothing to do while it seemed that everyone else was out having a ball, I cut my hair. It was just a whim. The next day a girl walked up to me and boldly said, "You fool!!" I couldn't understand her attitude. All my life, all I ever wanted was to be just like everybody else. Though people said I had "good hair," it didn't make me feel very good.

When Jessica was placed with me, her foster mother had been brushing her hair, adding only an occasional bow for adornment to distinguish Jessica from the baby boys that the woman also cared for. I continued to groom Jessica's hair that same way until her baby-sitter pointed out that we had to start "training" my baby's hair. She told me that I would have to do more with Jessica's hair than I had anticipated. I followed her suggestions and pulled Jessica's hair tightly into two little ponytails. It wasn't long before the hair began to break along the hairline. She hated having her hair combed, and although I believed that if I persisted she would eventually become accustomed to it and stop crying, my father, the doting PaPa, protested that I was hurting her, and convinced me to give up.

During that first visit my father remarked to me that Jessica had a pretty face. I was puzzled why he singled out her face instead of simply saying that Jessica is pretty. It was the kind of compliment given to a woman who is obese. I suddenly inferred from his statement that Jessica's "pretty" face made up for her "ugly" hair. I challenged my father after this dawned on me, and naturally he denied it. Yet I have always suspected that my parents were immediately attracted to each other because they both had the basic requirements they were seeking: light brown skin—lighter than mine—and straight hair. They adhered to the standards of beauty held by black people that were so prevalent in the 1940s. To my father, Jessica's hair detracted from her appearance. No doubt he considered her warm brown skin a drawback, as well.

For a few years I continued with the two-Afro-puff style I had managed to perfect until the puffs were so large that Jessica began to resemble Walt Disney's Dumbo. I tried just one ponytail, but when I would pick her up from day care, the shorter hair that did not stay snugly in her ponytail holder would be sticking out all around her head. She looked "wired" compared to the other children at day care, whose hair was still intact from the neatly secured braids from that morning.

When I tried parting Jessica's shorter hair in the middle and did my imitation of lateral cornrows, Jessica reminded me of a tiny ram with antlers, since my braiding tended to be quite large and irregular. I was disappointed with the results of my styling efforts, but my biggest obstacle was Jessica's extreme defiance over having her hair combed. After a professionally applied relaxer caused Jessica's hair to break off disastrously, we tried braids using extensions. This style was easy and attractive, until it was time to have them replaced. Removing the braids caused even more breakage.

We continued to experiment with different styles. There was a relaxed, blow-dried 'do that she liked but I thought was a bit mature-looking, besides being hard to maintain for a young, active child. Then there was a style in which we braided the hair at night and undid the braids in the morning, giving her a cute, crinkly look. But it too was high-maintenance.

Through all the style changes, the breakage continued. Finally I decided to have Jessica's hair cut short and to start all over. At the salon, the stylist gave her a neat, "texturized" bob. Jessica kept a faint smile on her face as she nodded politely when the stylist asked her if she liked her new style. As we walked out of the salon and the door closed behind us, Jessica burst into tears. Now she was further than ever from the long hair that she'd dreamed of. Through the agonizing sobs on the way home, I simply held her hand. Eventually the sobs gave way to anger. At home, between spells of temper tantrums, desperate crying, and condemning me as conspiring against her, I began to get a deeper glimpse of Jessica's feelings about herself and my feelings about Jessica.

She told me I had taken away the most important thing about her—her hair, despite the terrible condition it had been in. With short hair, she saw herself as being ugly and unlikable. I began to ache for her. It was devastating to realize that I had in some way allowed her to develop a self-concept in which her worth was determined by the way she looked. I so much want Jessica to be a stronger, more confident person than I am, and I felt as if I had done such a miserable job. I had only made her more obsessed about some image that she could never obtain. I began to cry with her.

Later, I wrestled with my own emotions. Maybe I had not been able to totally abandon the bourgeois standards that my parents instilled in me, unknowingly merging them into the ideas I had for Jessica's appearance. Why couldn't I just let her hair be woolly and even wild, as long as it's thoroughly washed and conditioned? Isn't that enough? But I also have to take into account the huge peer pressure on Jessica in our Virginia Beach community and her own wants and needs. Jessica has made it clear to me that she does not like Afros or dreadlocks. And I cannot bear the thought of having to hurt her by imposing such a style, which meets few ten-year-old African-American girls' ideas of attractiveness.

As I watch Jessica approach puberty, I know there are even more difficult days ahead. I want to protect her and convince her that she is beautiful, no matter what her hairstyle. But I know that she is reluctant to trust the mirror that is the reflection in my eye.

KIDDIE CHEMICAL SERVICES

Many girls get their first relaxer by first grade. With retouching done every six weeks, can you imagine how much chemical has been absorbed into the bloodstream by high school? I'm real big on protecting the rights of a child, and I do think that [putting relaxers on a child's head] equals child abuse in many situations. There's nothing out there that protects the rights of the child when it comes to toxic chemicals and how they play into asthma and other health conditions. You can't give alcohol to kids legally, and I don't feel parents have the right to do anything to a child for the sake of beauty.

—Peggy Dillard Toone, natural hair-care pioneer

TENDERHEADED
Nikky Finney

I am
and have been
since they used to pass me around
by my three mule braids
like a bowl of briarberries
no one wanted to touch
but everyone wanted to see

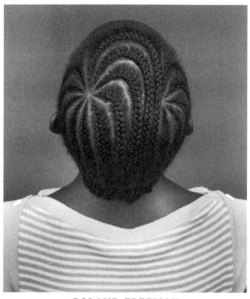

ROLAND FREEMAN

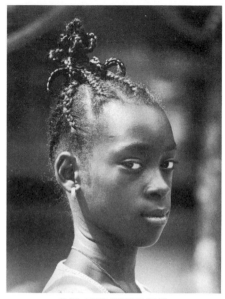

ROLAND FREEMAN

Darling Do's

"You take her!"
"Ohh no mam, I had her last time, remember?"

Nobody
Nobody
wanted to straighten this hair
and I didn't want nobody to

cotton mud brown and continent thick
they made bets on what color my scalp was
and how long it would take to get there
then would circle all around
hover over the swivel chair
just to know who had won
and who had lost

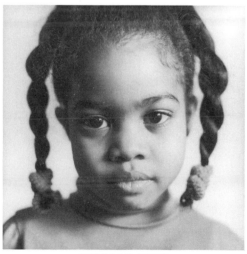

DEBORAH EGAN

easily
it was a day's travel
from the first to last sizzling stroke

afterward
whoever lost
politely walked over
and regretfully informed
the rest of her waiting customers
she was unavailable
for the rest of the day

while in the back room
already she was soaking her fingers
in a bowl of something sudsy and smooth
readying them
for their ordeal
and for the next four hours
I was hers

by large unsympathetic twisting fingers
she would take me
unmercifully
from chair to sink
to chair
to dryer
back to chair
and then finally
lead me up front near the window
just under the Clyburn's Beauty Shop sign
somewhere safe and faraway from those hands
where my scarlet and throbbing head

where my scorched ears
could cool better

behind me I could hear her
back with her girls now
her fingers returned to that sudsy bowl
waiting I suppose
for the color and the feeling to return
I could hear her
I could hear them all good
talking and teasing
about how the lord
must've got me mixed up
with somebody else
maybe even two or three people
giving me all that hair
and tenderheaded too

saying how some poor soul out on the street
right now walking around
with a big ole buffalo brush
and just a fingersnap of hair
steady pleading their mama or maybe even an auntie
for some squatting time inside that sacred place of places
and once inside those gaping legs how eyes would close
while hands scratched and brushed to high heaven
how they would sit so perfectly still
while their scalp got raked and planted
making sounds like they never wanted it to stop

still not knowing they so mismatched
not knowing maybe I got some of what belongs to them

just like them ladies don't know
how good I hear their laughter
ringing off the glass
that my head has made into
my cooling board
just like they don't know
how hard I'm trying not to hear them
how hard I'm steady peeping and looking outside
and longing for to get away
ride away
inside the safety of that '69 Buick
and back beside the generous giver of this
tenderheaded crown

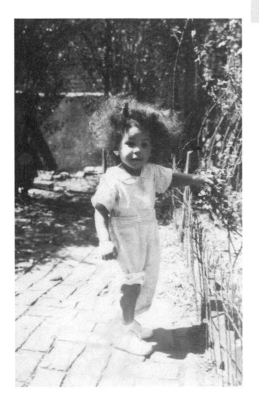

OH, SNAP!

How do you stop black children from jumping up and down on the bed?

Put Velcro on the ceiling.

This tiny soul sister in Harrisburg, PA, in 1946, is way ahead of her time with an early 1970s 'fro and 1990s one-pants-leg-rolled-up panache.

JULIETTE HARRIS COLLECTION

CORNROW CALCULATIONS (OR MATH IS BEAUTY)
Toni Wynn

Word to the Reader: The first part of this essay is so true that the second part vibed onto the page just to affirm all of the remarkable stuff Dr. Gilmer told me.

—Your reporter

I

Gloria Gilmer looks at the triangles, squares, parallels, and zigzag lines on black girls' and men's heads—where most cornrows can be found these days—and sees mathematical principles as well as art. Convinced that the design strategies of braiders can be used to interest young people in math, Gilmer, an educational consultant, has carved out an area of mathematics devoted to developing cornrow curricula.

Looking back at her journey through life, Gloria Gilmer, who holds mathematics degrees from Morgan State and the University of Pennsylvania and a Ph.D. in curriculum and instruction from Marquette University, sees stepping stones from her childhood up to her present mission. The youngest of three, she was raised in Baltimore by the book—the Good Book and the math book. Her minister had a master's degree in mathematics from the University of Pennsylvania and folks at her Episcopal church were her algebra and calculus teachers. "Math was all tied up with my religion," Gilmer says. "I understood the mathematics first, then I understood the essential nature of human beings from the mathematical structures." In other words, there are patterns in numbers and patterns in our bodies.

From age nine, Gloria worked at her father's store after school and on weekends, applying her math skills. She preferred subtraction over addition and division over multiplication because "you can check your work. It feels very powerful to have a way, on your own, to find out if you're right. You become sure of yourself."

Gilmer is one of the originators of "ethnomathematics," the study of a cultural group's interaction with math. Fractals, a new kind of geometry, led Gilmer to study design patterns in black folk's hair. Her discussion of "Hairstyles in

African American Communities" drew an overflow crowd at a National Council of Teachers of Mathematics conference. The purpose of her work is to attract the community to the discipline of mathematics, which, she, observes, "has really ignored my people." She feels strongly that public education should be more relevant to the cultures of the students and that most of the current math instruction is "too dull."

Gilmer's research assistant, Stephanie, is a fifteen-year-old New York high school student with Haitian roots. The two go into beauty parlors looking for patterns in hair braiding, then analyze the embedded mathematical ideas. She instructs her protégée to look closely at the scalp, because, she says, "That's where the action is."

Gilmer taught college math for many years before establishing Math-Tech, an educational consulting business in Milwaukee. She's been speaking out about ethnomathematics since the early 1980s. But whether she's on a campus, in a corporate boardroom or at Maxi's NuVogue beauty shop, one unwavering purpose guides Gloria Gilmer's way: "I have a passion for justice. Wherever I'm working, it's always about justice."

II

Gloria Gilmer's passion is embodied in Princess Tesselation, a girl who always uses her cornrowed head. Come along on the Math-Is-Beauty Tour! Princess Tesselation is the guide, and I'm your reporter. Let's get ready for the journey. . . .

Left brain aligned with right? Check.

Tape recorder, camera, phone? Check.

Calculator? Oh, yeah. Almost forgot that.

The Muse? Beauty. Beauty stepping on the main stage, where education is. Beauty from work, moving with power. Don't be afraid to do the math, it helps you look good.

Affirmation: I look at Beauty, and she's an invitation to deeper mysteries/a language of signs, like math. And spirit: She cooks breakfast each morning served as prayer. Knowing her is a lease, a toehold on joy. She and Power almost look the same: silent, brushing each other's hair. Beauty is freedom from doubt.

Vibe? Knowledge. Believe it. *Estamos listas.*

We're rolling now.

How did Princess Tess get her name?

Tesselations are beautiful patterns of interlocking forms, with no spaces between. (No room for doubt.) Tesselation is useful. Box braids and triangle braids are good examples. A rectangular tesselation of the scalp uses a pattern we recognize from bricklaying. You see, hairstyles and mathematics are natural partners.

Math is everywhere you look. Quilters, bankers, athletes, architects, seamstresses, and hair braiders all use mathematical ideas. There's trigonometry in basketball and pool; algebra in getting from your house to mine; and fractal geometry in cornrows. You following me? Fractals describe, mathematically of course, systems in the human body that have patterns like plants such as trees and ferns, which have branches that grow ever smaller. That's like braids getting smaller towards the end.

THE MAKING OF A ROAD SCHOLAR

Princess Tesselation and her people are up all night making ready for the tour. Godparents, philosophers, beauticians, the tutor, financial adviser, advance man, and a pantheon of other royalty—Princesses Science, Literature and Arts and Princes Humanities and Technology—all extended family. Even the stuffed animals are up, wired in fuzziness. Somebody finally admonishes our girl, "Tesselate yourself some sleep so you'll make some kind of sense to all those people tomorrow!"

Princess Tess knew early on that she was meant for this ambassadorship, this license to inspire. She loves to know and share. She listens well, too. When ethnomathematics was introduced during a black history month program, Tess was quick to call the salons and e-mail her math teacher. She is an activist, and the time is always now.

First stop, Teaneck, New Jersey.

Sound check.

Princess Tess clips on the body mike. She is beauty multiplied by power in stretch khakis, a yellow T-shirt with a big orange pi symbol denoting the ratio of the circumference of a circle to its diameter silk-screened on the front, a fresh pedicure, and zigzag-parted cornrows emanating from a circular part on top of her head out of which a lone braid sprouts and curves back into an arc.

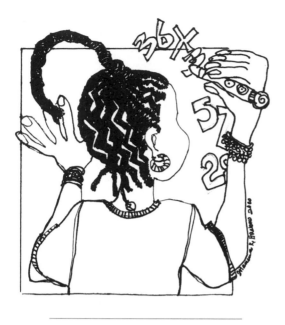

Princess Tess doing cornrow calculations.

FRANCINE HASKINS

Here she is:

Can you all hear me in the back? They call me Princess Tesselation, but my friends call me Tess.

(Kujichagulia energy clicks in!)

I'll just talk for a bit so you guys can get your sound levels, OK? Now, when I was a kid I didn't really care what my hair looked like. We'd just pull it back and let it explode or stick straight out on the other side of the scrunchie. And I was not available to sit in somebody's chair for five hours. But then I turned thirteen, and stuff was beginning to matter. All the lip gloss and eyebrow shaving in the world couldn't take the place of the right hair. So who do you think came along? Dr. Gilmer! I heard about ethnomath and decided to try cornrows, even though I knew my brother would probably start calling me Spree because of Latrell Sprewell. But I didn't care as long as it would further my education and keep me looking good at the same time. Then, everything started happening at once, and now I'm famous. And my friends are trying to be royalty along with me. I tell them sure they can, if they know their math!

After a rousing speech, Princess Tess slips into the mathmobile, brightly painted with numbers, symbols and fractals, and is whisked off to her next appearance.

A chanting, multi-culti crowd has gathered. The mood is Rio in Dar es Salaam in central Jersey. The theme is pattern and rhythm. They form a rumba line.

"Princess Tess a lay SHUN!"

"Princess Tess a lay SHUN!"

A small plane cruises low over the community, trailing a banner. It reads:

$$S = 2+3+4...+n= [(9n+2)(n-1)]/2$$

The man with the headset counts back from five, four, three, two, gives the cue. Tess looks up at the sky and says:

Given: S = the number of braids, and N = the number of rows + 1.

That is, given you know what cornrows are.

Everybody laughs and breaks out their calculators!

Hi, this is Tess! I'm glad you came out today so I can tell you about the work that Dr. Gloria Gilmer is doing. She is real and she wants us to be aware and financially comfortable. Everybody here wants us to be beautiful and we know how power comes right along with that so here is the truth: I have Dr. Gilmer in my head at all times and she is funny but totally serious.

Look how wonderfully my braids are tesselated and I get A's in math all the time. Every time I go to study hall people crowd all around me wanting to learn from my hair. They're all, "Tess, bend your head down so I can do exponents. Stand in the light so we can study the patterns."

No matter what, Dr. Gilmer is with me. I've got to know math; it builds my leadership skills. It makes me smarter. At least I feel that way.

When somebody asks me out, they always say I'm beautiful and I don't even get embarrassed anymore because I feel it too, and I'm not trying to brag or anything, but the more you know and the more you can do, the more beauty and power become part of your life.

Preach!

Like check this out: Do you want your hair to move a lot or a little? Here's something I learned from ethnomath. When hair strands within a triangle are brought to the center, the braids are less likely to swing. But braids formed by bringing hair strands to the bottom point of the triangle to a vertex will move when your head moves. This is happening on our heads, everybody. We are Living Tesselations! Truth is beauty! Tesselate on!

Tess's court works the crowd until every hand holds a neon yellow flyer illustrated with equations and pictures of famous braided heads. The flyer reads:

Cornrows are mathematics for the eyes. From deep culture to the classroom. What's on the head serves inside the head. The natural connection of mathematics with braids is Beautiful.

We don't have to run out of hair before the job is done.

We can know how long the job will take.

Applied ethnomath. Ujamaa to the bone!

Call toll-free 1 888 555 TESS for the hookup!

Tess's tutor, a biracial woman whose 178 braids all spring out at the bottom, takes to the top of the stoop on the last stop of the day. She is moved to connect with the hair braiders in the crowd and beyond. She rocks the mike like she's at a poetry slam. . . .

If I see your hands flying through my child's hair and I'm holding your baby and the telephone is silent and the television is not on, can we talk about what you're doing? It starts out regular, then whoops, turns science fiction—the range of your skills is fantastic. The geography of the head—you the cartographer negotiating roads through these thickets. We get to art (go ahead and smile), which is where you were coming from anyway. Then uh oh, you're at math, using an ancient matrix and twenty-first century knowledge to make bank. I pay you well because you know how it's done in formulas/soulscape/exchange, living for living.

A power move putting braids in hair. A path to beauty. Using the tools, the braider with sweet breath and some laughter crowns a new queen. Power glimmers, glides into vision for seeing more, seeing deeper. We know the promise of infinity and you are the Plus One. We have learned well the false statements of "far enough" and have been complacent in the absence of leaders.

(Then the tutor thinks about all the salons she's visited and all exploitation because the women don't do the math.)

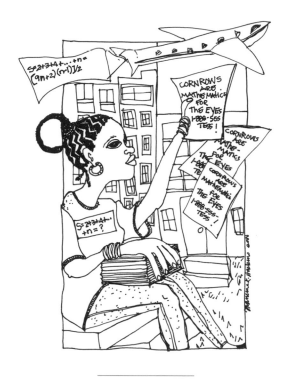

Princess Tess on the stoop.

FRANCINE HASKINS

"Oh no, girl, I don't mess with no math, I just do hair make change keep the stuff I need in the back so I don't have to have somebody run out when I need something. Oh no, girl I stay away from math I just balance my books pay my vendors tesselate some hair. What did I just say? I don't recognize that word. Must be some fairies in here.

"Look at those double dutch queens outside in the parking lot, can't nobody get by them. They're jumping triple time now. I been watching them for years. Helps my fingers keep moving. Oh no, girl I can't take it no farther than running a business and tesselating some tenderheads as I sleepwalk through knowing. I read in the paper every day about all I don't know."

Stand up!

We are, still and now, diffused, needing gurus, griots, intermediaries to mentor us in beauty. What our responsibilities might be. How to do math. How to write success in the languages we speak. Step aboard the Princess Tess mathmobile. Not only can we give you that day-spa glow, but your power is ensured. Next stop, a stoop you know. Thanks for coming!

Store-Bought Hair

*W*hen it comes to keeping up appearances, the contemporary black woman has a warehouse full of options. She's got weaves, wigs, extensions, pieces, puffs, and pin-on ponytails. She can get them in colors ranging from blond to blue to burgundy, and set them off with chopsticks, rhinestone bobby pins, fluttering butterfly barrettes, with plenty more Goodys to spare. The sky used to be the limit, but sistergirl crashed through that a long time ago.

WAIT! I HAVE AN IDEA!

Seen at a Detroit Hair Wars show, one of several of its kind around the country: A man in a Superman-style get-up known as the Super Hair Fighter; a short blond cut with animal-print spots; plastic dog bones adorning the curls of an updo; and, a man turning a model into a vase for a two-foot plant made of hair.

—From *The Detroit Free Press,* 2000

FAKE

Gerrie Summers

It was the late eighties and a friend and I were at yet another listening party for a hip-hop group. As she and I talked and sipped our drinks, a young rap producer we both knew walked up and started playing with my friend's long, thick mane.

"I like your hair," he said, stroking it softly. "You know why?"

■ 3000–1596 B.C. ■

ANCIENT WIGDOMS

For almost 3,000 years there was little variation in hairstyling in Egypt! Egyptian women first wore their own hair braided and decorated with shells, glass, and other items. Then, between 3000 and 1596 B.C., the Egyptians moved from wearing natural braids to favoring wigs. "Women cut their hair very short and wore wigs made of sheep's wool, because it was closest to their natural texture. Flax or palm-fibre were also used to create wigs, and examples were found in early tombs."

—Victoria Wurdinger, *The Multicultural Client: Cuts, Styles, and Chemical Services*

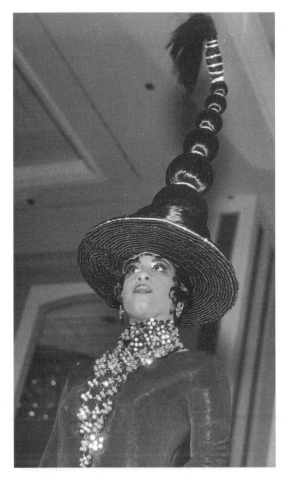

HIGH NUBIAN STYLE

During the eighteenth dynasty, Egyptians went from wearing long wigs to short wigs as a result of the influence of their Queen Tiye, a black woman of Nubian ancestry. A photograph of a bust of Tiye shows the dark-brown-skinned queen with hair in a style that today would be called a medium-length Afro with a high top.

—Christiane Desroches-Noblecourt, *Tutankhamen: Life and Death of a Pharaoh*

"Don't Be Afraid of Heights"
Proud Lady Hair & Beauty Show
Chicago, Illinois, 1994.

BILL GASKINS

"No, why?" she asked, feigning interest because she'd heard this line from him before.

"Because it's real."

More than a compliment to her, I felt his comment was meant as an insult to me. At the time, I wore long, braided extensions, and some of the brothers had decided that this hairstyle made me a fake and therefore open to ridicule. They asserted that somehow, wearing a hairpiece proved that a woman was ashamed of who she was. Or that she was trying to be somebody that she was not. But to me, the stream of put-downs were simply another way for black men, who often feel powerless in this society, to punish someone—namely black women—and for things *we* have no control over, like the clash between our hair and mainstream standards of beauty. God, I was so tired of this!

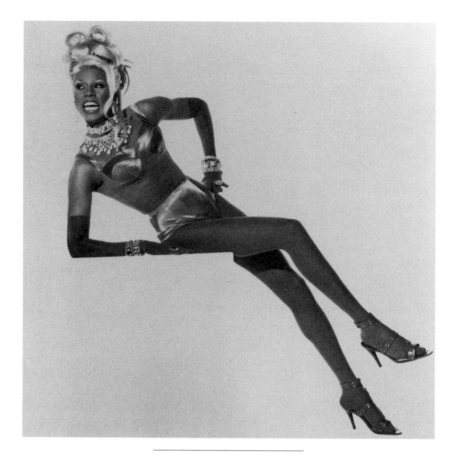

RuPaul: The Ultimate Makeover.

PHOTOFEST

My friend's hair, by the way, just happened to be a *real* good weave. Perhaps no one realized it because the hair was not bone straight. But what if the young rap producer had discovered the truth? Would my friend no longer be worthy of his admiration? Would she, like little ol' extension-wearing me, be, God forbid, a fake? Just who was real and who was bogus in that situation?

During that time, I edited *Word Up*, a hip-hop publication that featured mostly young male rappers. Ours was the first national publication to give them major play. Most black magazines at the time seemed reluctant to cover this new music form, since it went against black middle-class sensibilities. It was too loud and too vulgar, they argued. Now, I wasn't crazy about this urban street sound myself, but I had readers to please. And slowly, some of the records actually began to grow on me. The performers didn't have as many attitude problems back then, either. Although they became notorious for outbursts of bad behavior a decade later, most of the artists in the mid-eighties treated me with respect.

Back then, I gave hip-hop props as well for getting scores of young men and women—who probably would have wound up in juvenile detention, pregnant, or on the streets—a way out of poverty and crime. Rap ruled the airwaves, its jargon invaded the nation's vocabulary, street gear took over the fashion world, and the culture influenced Madison Avenue. Even the Pillsbury Doughboy was dropping some rhymes.

But there was a downside.

Rap was an extremely sexist genre that included few female artists. Many young male rappers spewed misogynistic insults into the mike. At first they referred to women as "skeezers" and "hoes," and then went on to include newly coined terms such as "fake-hair-wearin' bitch," which condemned black women for the sin of wearing weaves and extensions.

I was already struggling with featuring rap acts that I found offensive, such as 2 Live Crew, but I held on to the hope that I could change some of these performers' Neanderthal attitudes through the pages of the magazine. But the powers-that-be saw only dollar signs, not the pain that the music caused women like me. With the advent of gangster rap and more violent lyrics toward women and the world in general, I would later resign.

The barrage of attacks on black women with fake hair made me livid, especially since most white women with blond hair really aren't blondes, and many with curly hair got it out of a box. It's a given that a white woman can change her hair for style, but too often a black woman's desire to change her look is deemed an affront to the race.

When I was growing up in the sixties and seventies, I didn't have many options for styling my hair, so I attempted to straighten it with home relaxer kits. They never worked on my coarse hair, and left it even more difficult to style. Later, with an array of braided options to choose from, I gladly abandoned the chemicals that had ravaged my hair for years. But when I chose to wear styles that called for extensions, did I forfeit my right to be respected?

A hip-hop publicist I worked with at that time told me he believed the hair-insult wave in rap was a crossover from R&B—specifically, in fact, from the 1987 song "Fake," by soul-crooner Alexander O'Neal. "Your hair was long," he sang, "but now it's short. You said, 'I cut it off,' but I don't see no hair on the floor." Then he goes on to give his girl a litany of reasons why she's a fake, and he's through with her.

The song was a huge hit, and—as is the norm in the recording industry—everyone jumped on the bandwagon. Working a hair joke into a conversation, skit, or rhyme became the thing to do. Comedians jumped on it with four feet. And a one-hit-wonder group called Bobby Jimmy and the Critters followed up with a silly record called "Hair or Weave," a takeoff on the R&B group Today's "Him or Me."

During that time, you were hard-pressed to listen to a rap album without being subjected to at least one rhyme slamming fake hair. For a genre that thrives on the put-down, it was perfect. Some of it was funny. Most of it was not.

References to hair became yet another way to prey upon the insecurities of black women. I began to wonder, How many of these black men harbor a deep-seated resentment of black women? How many brothers actually *long* for the flowing manes that become repugnant to them only when they learn they are not real? I contend that the frequent protest against extensions and weaves so prevalent in rap rhymes had less to do with blackness or even being fake than with giving men another weapon to dehumanize women.

Men have always objectified women to soothe the wounds of rejection. To be rejected by a woman you're interested in is a blow to the heart, but to be dissed by an object you merely wanted for sex is a minor flesh wound. A cutting remark about extensions or weaves gave men the perfect comeback to a rebuff by a woman who was wearing one. One of the most offensive attacks came from the rap group No Face, featuring 2 Live Crew. The track, called "Fake Hair Wearin' Bitch," smacks of retaliation by a man who feels belittled by a woman who looks down on him "like I ain't shit." And what better, more mature way to punish her than to attack her hair: "Yes, I'm dissin' when I say Bitch, you need some fuckin' help to find out who you really are. . . . Your hair ain't real / Don't think I don't know the deal."

Counterattacks came from women who were tired of being passed over for the long-haired types. On "I've Been Watchin' You for a While," Father MC raps with Lady Kazan, who doesn't believe him for a minute.

"Don't even bother," she says.

"Why not?" he responds.

"I think your personality stinks."

"Just because I offered to buy you a drink?"

"Don't even try it. You didn't think I saw you over there / Rapping with the girl with the long, fake hair?"

The eighties concept of "keeping it real" went beyond the no-weaves, no-Jheri-curls, no-blue-contact-lens mandate. It also involved knowing where you came from, staying true to the streets, and being down with your homeboys. The artist called Sound from the group Zhigge put it this way in "Born Black": "I'll stomp a blue contact or curl without a doubt / Keep my hair dreaded because you know I ain't no sellout."

At the close of the eighties and into the nineties, the conviction grew among some that hair, physical features, and a certain code of behavior held the power to define blackness. The times gave rise to several Afrocentric artists. One, King Sun, attacked many of the bandwagon pro-black rappers whose knowledge of self was, in his estimation, lacking and untrue. But there was pure irony in his rhyme, "Be Black," in which he berates women who are "hard as calluses instead of being sweet, truthful and soft / They want to be fake, and that turns me off." He criticizes their synthetic hair and unusual eye colors while acknowledging his preference for "redbone" (i.e., light-skinned) women. If King Sun is puzzled why women are, as he put it, "callous," his lyrics should provide him a clue. He faults black women for altering their hair or features and, in nearly the same breath, states a preference for black women with these same European features.

On a track called, "Extensions," the hip-hop group Stetsasonic got in an equally nasty swipe at the sisters: "Here's something we should mention / Bald-headed girls with extensions / Here's something we think you should know / Listen up, it might make the hair grow." The message was that there is ignorance behind a desire to wear extensions or weaves and that the "educated" brothers were going to harrass, ridicule, and bully black women back to their natural state. Fortunately, one cooler head prevailed. On "Around the Way Girl," L. L. Cool J decided to "dedicate at least one rhyme" to all the cuties in the neighborhood. He went on to celebrate a range of women with a wide spectrum of hair styles: "I wanna girl with extensions in her hair," he rapped, later giving a nod as well to the homegirl with "a perm in your hair, even a curly weave." Unlike many male artists who sought out drop-dead gorgeous, longer-haired lovers, L. L. Cool J's taste in women transferred from wax to real life. His girlfriend, who became his wife, had a girl-next-door beauty and shorter hair.

Over the years, I've noticed that I've received more looks and compliments from men when I've worn my braids long than when I've worn them short. And I've seen women with long hair—however it was connected to their heads—consistently get the man, the job, and the rap-video role.

All brouhaha aside, the constant barrage of insults from the rap world hasn't put a dent in the hair trade. And the technology has become so sophisticated that a skilled weaver can add in extra hair, making the site of the attachment invisible even to the most scrutinizing eye. Weaves are now done several ways: the braided technique where the natural hair is cornrowed and the weave is sewn onto the row; bonding, in which the weave is glued onto your hair; and French lacing, in which loose hair is braided into cornrows and the ends are left free. In fact, you can even achieve the locks it took Bob Marley years to grow in a single afternoon—with the help of extensions. I've noticed that it's harder for men to poke fun at *these* extensions, since so many of them now wear them.

In her song "Doo Wop (That Thing)," Lauryn Hill called out fake women *and* men who say one thing yet do another: "Let it sit inside your head like a million women in Philly, Penn," she rapped. "It's silly when girls sell their souls because it's in / Look at where you be in hair weaves like Europeans / Fake nails done by Koreans." And she adds a verse for the man who is "more concerned with his rims [wheels] and his Timbs [boots] than his women." These days, however, it is increasingly difficult to define what's real in hip-hop when so many rappers are hanging out with Hollywood shot-callers or chillin' in traditionally lily-white vacation havens. What would be considered fake in the eighties is now prized. Materialism is in. And so, apparently, are women of mixed heritage with long, straight hair. I guess you might say they are *real* exotic.

As far as I can see, this battle is far from over, as "We Both Frontin'," a track from the rapper Mase's 1999 *Harlem World* CD, illustrates. On it, a brother spots a young lady with a pretty smile, "a real fine queen / eyes were light green," who is half Haitian and half Asian. The queen, however, isn't interested since the

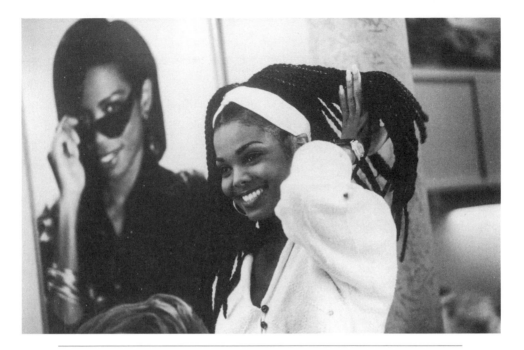

Janet Jackson works the hair and the nails for her role in the 1993 movie Poetic Justice.

PHOTOFEST

watch on the man's wrist doesn't contain real jewels: "I like that platinum on your wrist / But why is there no ice in this?" she asks. His answer: "Same reason why, baby girl, that ain't your hair. We both frontin'."

IN OTHER WORDS . . .

HORSE HAIR: The synthetic hair that is generally used in weaves and wigs. Stick-straight and unnaturally glossy, this hair is the hallmark of a very bad weave. "Doll's hair wig" connotes the same thing.

▪ 1914 ▪

The "father of the blues," W. C. Handy, knew how one black woman's counterfeit hair could be another woman's heartache. He captured it in the classic song "St. Louis Woman": "If it weren't for powder and all that store-bought hair / That man of mine wouldn't have gone nowhere."

OH, SNAP!

From the stage, popular comic Somemore, who has been known to wear her hair in a bob, cracked on fellow comedian Thea, seated nearby and wearing long, flowing blond hair: "Thea said she ain't goin' back to Africa 'cause there's nobody there that can do her weave."

"I used to wear a weave myself," Somemore quipped. "When I got rid of my fake hair, I stopped attracting fake men."

PLANET HAIR
Lisa Jones

I haven't read J. A. Rogers's *100 Amazing Facts about the Negro* yet, so I wonder if it tells of any amazing triumphs over Bad Hair. Like our patron saint of Good Hair, Madam C. J. Walker, who made a small fortune off the scalps of Negro women who had so little time to "Fix that Mess" (as a recent ad for Le Kair's Black Satin Cream Relaxer says). Or of the incredible balancing acts of Tamara Dobson ("Run your fingers through my nine-inch 'fro if you want to, daddy, I got a gun to your jugular") and Miss Ross ("I need twelve inches or more").

Is there mention of Harlem's Hair Station on 125th Street (owned by Koreans, Rogers would have pointed out)? Or of its manager, Alexis Smith, a black man who for the past nine years has made his living putting that heifer Mother Nature in her place?

▪ 1993 ▪

WE'VE ALWAYS WORN WEAVES!

At a symposium at the University of Delaware art historian Judith Wilson links African-American women's hair straightening, extensions, wigs, and weave wearing to a principle in traditional African aesthetics that she calls "antinaturalism." Referring to sub-Saharan African practices that lengthen and expand the volume of curly hair (such as coating the hair with mud or adding animal hair, feathers, beads, or fibers to it), Wilson maintains that along with "a preference for *abundance,* then, both Africans and African American hair styles frequently exhibit a high degree of *artifice.* Indeed, where Western culture generally condemns most forms of body adornment or alteration as vain, deceitful, grotesque, tasteless, or at best merely frivolous, Africans tend to view *failure* to supplement, transform, or otherwise improve on nature as a lapse of character or a breach of decorum."

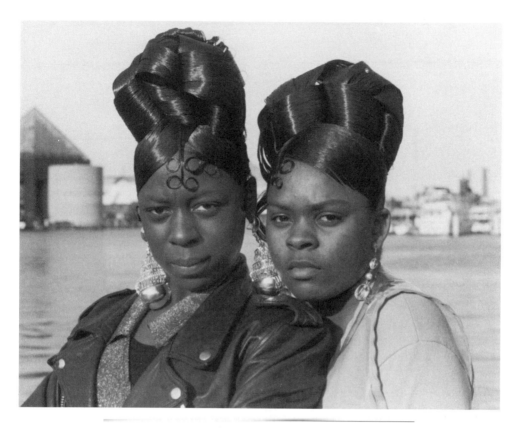

Tamara and Tarika, Easter Sunday, Baltimore, Maryland, 1995.

BILL GASKINS

It's a just-got-paid Friday, just after five. You can see the sign from Lenox Avenue:

Hair Station
Manufacture
100% Human Hair
Braiding & Weaving

Near the IRT entrance on Lenox and 125th, Rastas selling bootleg shearling are blasting Marley's "Could You Be Loved" ("Don't let them change you / Or

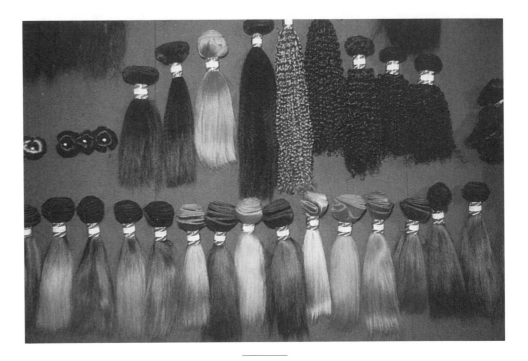

The Goods.

ALLFORD/TROTMAN

even rearrange you / Oh no"). The sounds trail down the block to Hair Station's small storefront, where hair, real human hair, hangs in neatly coiffed horsetails from every inch of wall space. Some is displayed, like scalps, in glass cases.

The after-work crowd works the counters. A half dozen young women in black shearling (real) and leather (real) hover over one counter petting a length of "Bone Straight." (Which may take its name from the new relaxer by TCB. "Not just straight," the ads promise, "Bone Straight.") They compare it to "French Refined" ("European stock," bouncy, silky, with a hint of curl), which Alexis says is tied with "Bone Straight" for best-seller: " 'Bone Straight' is hot right now, but the most versatile hair out is 'French Refined.' It doesn't condemn you to one style."

CAUCASIAN STRAIGHT, KINKY STRAIGHT, KINKY AFRO

Whose hair was this before? Hair Station imports it in bulk, mostly from Asia, where poor women sell their long, straight locks for money. The hair is "re-textured" in a secret heating process ("bogus places use chemicals," says Alexis) to match black hair types, permed, Jheri curled, or untreated.

"There's Chinese hair and hair from Italy," adds the Korean owner, a stocky man who asks not to be identified. "The European hair is more expensive because it's rare. One or two people a year come to us off the street to sell their hair, some Spanish girls, but we can't do that. That little amount doesn't help us."

You choose from unlimited blends of brown, black, and blond, or novelty colors like neon yellow (Phyllis Diller), deep purple (circa George Clinton's Brides of Funkenstein), and siren red (Chaka Khan). "We don't dye like everyone else," Alexis confides. "We have a secret way of dyeing."

PRICES ARE SUBJECT TO CHANGE WITHOUT NOTICE

"Price depends on texture and color," Alexis will tell you. "I got hair, twenty-two bucks, good hair. Places try to sell you the lower-quality stuff for more money. Buy bad hair, after a couple days, it tangles, it itches. If you sweat, the chemicals go to your scalp.

"Big-time salons, downtown and Fifth Avenue, buy our hair. They condition it before they do the weaves or the braids and charge their clients two and three grand. Places in California make it four or five."

WEAVING THREADS AND NEEDLES SOLD

Alexis holds up to my temple the most expensive item in the store, a thirty-inch auburn length of "Kinky Straight." It passes my knees. The owner nudges Alexis in the ribs. "Tell her about the bald ladies with the bald hair. That's funny. They don't want to show it to you."

Alexis explains: "Women come in, you know what they need, everybody knows what they need. But you have to find a way to tell them, without saying your hair is bald, whatever. Without offending them. Because people are very offended. Their hair is thin."

What would you say to a woman who doesn't have a lot of hair? That she needs a wig?

"No!"

The faux pas is mine. Wigs, you see, to a midwife of manes like Alexis, are a last resort, a lazy way out. "There are many different methods of weaving or braiding hair in." Alexis counts off on his fingers as if addressing a group of preschoolers. "You can glue it in, you can sew it in, do box braids. There's a new system called interlocks. It's so good, a guy could run his fingers through your hair and nothing could happen."

HEADS WITH HUMAN HAIR AVAILABLE TO BEAUTY SCHOOL

Let me ask you this, I say to Alexis. Some people say, uhm, some people think, that it's not right for black women to wear hair, you know, weaves, and maybe they should just wear their own hair and be natural. What do you think about that? Uh, the politics of that?

Alexis rolls his eyes. "Most women who buy hair for weaving actually don't have hair. It's the convenience of it. If the weave enhances them in the process, so be it. By all means use the hair. But if the black man really likes you, he's gonna like you for you, not because of your weave."

SUPER WAVY, EUROPEAN WAVY, KINKY AFRO

A mature woman in Blackglama mink slaps Alexis's cheek when he tries to have a look under her matching hat. He can only smile.

"Me dealing with women, I really understand. When you wake up every morning and you gotta hot curl, press, comb everything, and go to work? It's not gonna happen.

"My customers see guys walking past the door and they go 'AAAAAyyyye!'" Alexis hides his face in his hands. "But me, they don't care. When I first started working here I was like a male looking in. You're coming to a whole new world. I can't say I'm a woman now, but I got a pass card."

DEEP WAVY, BODY WAVY, JHERI CURL

This is a blood bank. Hair types A, AA, B. Bad hair, warns Alexis, the kind that Hair Station doesn't sell, the kind tainted with chemicals that irritate the scalp, is a bad transfusion.

"They sell low-quality hair all over the city," Alexis tells me. "Places have even started carrying the yak hair, which is animal hair."

You mean they try to pass it off as human hair?

"Yeah, yeah, this is New York," says Alexis. "I won't get egotistical and say we sell the best hair in the city, but we're the leaders. When we deal with hair, it's a personal thing. Our customers trust us like they trust their doctors."

It's almost seven now. With fifteen minutes to closing, women pack the store so there's scarce breathing room. They push between counters in search of the perfect weekend piece. A young woman in purple shearling pounds on a display case, her sights on a length of "Bone Straight" protected behind glass.

They forbid me to come back Saturday. Alexis keeps shaking his head: "It's a madhouse." I want to stay behind the counter some more with Alexis. Watch him watch us get close to the mirror,

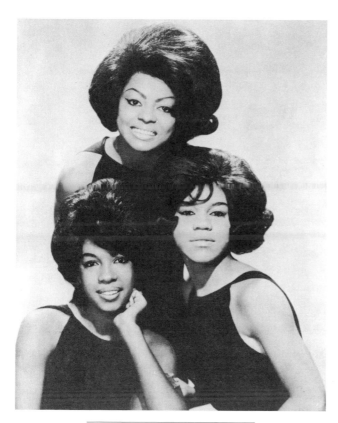

The Supremes wiggled through the 1960s.

PHOTOFEST

real close, painful close. Like this: You hold a length of hair up to your face, and you squint. Give us profile, straight on, squint some more. Picture your man's hands in your hair or "hair that moves" (says an ad for TCB No Lye Relaxer) or fifteen minutes of extra time in the morning. Then Alexis saunters over; he's not here to play you. And when the time is right, when you've decided, *really* decided, he sends you home, with the real you, wrapped up neatly in a brown paper bag.

HAIR TO THERE

There isn't a single art supply store in all of Newark. I am drawn into a beauty supply shop, one of the few thriving businesses in the city. Flowing from display after display, a plethora of hair of any description: smooth, real, synthetic, black, off black, blond or red, kenkalon, braided, straight or curly. All for sale. As much as any black girl could ever dream of. . . .

Artist Eve Sandler recalls the period when she lived in a loft in an abandoned factory in Newark. The profusion of hair in the shop inspired her to use it as a medium. *Hair to There,* an installation consisting of long hanks of synthetic hair, was exhibited in 1997 at the Rush Art Gallery in New York City. The installation was part of the artist's High Maintenance series, which examines issues of femininity that are "particularly loaded for black women," says Sandler.

Describing black women's use of long synthetic hair and fanglike fingernails as "incredibly complex," the artist says that *Hair to There* reflects "a paradox of Eurocentric desire wrapped up in African-inspired traditions." Contending that the desire for long hair is not just about wanting to look white, Sandler explains that in Africa hair and nails are used in masks to "extend the boundaries of the female body to near surreal lengths."

"In working with [synthetic hair]," she explains, "I seek to communicate the inherent

---

▪ 1970 ▪

FAMOUS LAST WORDS

In the moments leading up to the 1970 farewell performance of Diana Ross and the Supremes, before La Ross went solo, the girls were buzzing about the dressing room of the Frontier Hotel in Las Vegas: "Pass me your lipstick," Mary Wilson says to Cindy Birdsong. "Are you wearing that curly wig tonight? I sure wish I'd brought my blond wig. . . ."

—from *Supreme Faith,*
Mary Wilson

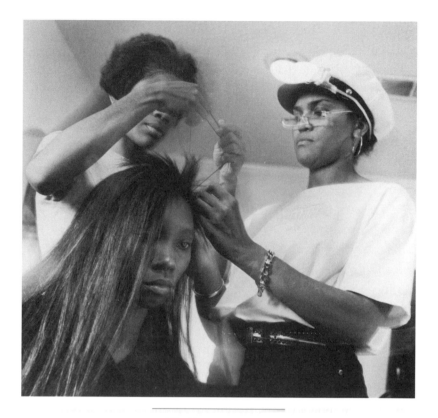

Hooking up a weave.

ALLFORD/TROTMAN

power and tradition in ritualized extensions of self even as I wonder what too long might be."

HAIR BRAIDING, MISS?
Taiia Smart

All along Harlem's 125th Street, West African women catch my eye, asking softly, "Hair braiding, Miss?" They huddle in twos and threes near the subway entrances, at the bus stops, near the portals of their storefronts. I pass by quickly, usually on my way somewhere else, but always curious about the women whose colorful print dresses and hopeful faces stay with me. Then one day, I befriend one of the sisters, asking if I may follow her to her shop to watch.

Fatima* works at Mains D'Or, one of the most popular African braiding sa-lons in upper Manhattan. It is located at the top of a narrow, meandering stair-case. And since it's Saturday, the joint is jumping. Ten stylists are scattered be-tween the two adjoining rooms, and clumps of faux hair dot the floor. Fussing over heads, the stylists quote prices for braid work about to begin or spray clouds of oil sheen on heads that are just being completed. The charge is $39 for flat twists (twists that lay flat against the scalp) and $100 for box braids. These same styles would cost more in New Jersey and Connecticut, but on this block compe-tition "inspires" reasonable prices.

Like a Varnette Honeywood painting, chocolate, mocha, and vanilla-hued faces line the perimeter of the shop. Their expressions reflect the restlessness that comes with the long waits, and yet they all have 'dos in varying needs of repair. They pass the time bopping their heads to the beats pumping in their Walk-mans, reading novels, or perusing the current issues of a half-dozen black hair magazines, searching for last-minute ideas. Fatima, a beautiful, cinnamon-colored woman with her own micro braids swept up in a French roll, is perched on a stool. She gives the woman before her box braids, rapidly entwining real hair with synthetic strands pulled from a long, cellophane bag. She's been at it for hours. Exhausted, she bends her neck to the side as she repeats the process: Part a small box in the scalp, braid the section to the end, and then flick on a lighter, letting the tiny orange flame singe the braid's tip, melting it like plastic, so it won't unravel.

A few years ago, when Fatima, along with her husband Amadou, arrived here from Senegal, she knew nothing about braiding. Back home, some women went to salons to have their hair braided but mainly did each other's heads. In America, however, Fatima saw big money in braiding. Eager to ditch her cashier's job at a local supermarket, she learned the business from a girlfriend who owns three shops in Brooklyn. She observed the friend at work and often helped out doing box braids. The first time Fatima styled hair without her men-tor's assistance, however, she could hardly get through it.

"I was shaking and sweating," Fatima recalls in her West African lilt. Still,

---

*Some names and identifying details have been changed to protect the subjects' privacy.

everything turned out all right with the goddess-braid hairstyle. "The braid that wrapped around her head wasn't really in the center, but she liked it anyway."

Since then, Fatima's collected lots of hair stories, like the time she earned a $50 tip. ("I kept it for a week before I spent it.") Or when an admirer of her work followed one of her clients around a beach in Jamaica, snapped a picture of her braids, and requested Fatima's phone number. The thirty-three-year-old mother tells these stories matter-of-factly, yet her cheeks beam with pride.

Then there are the ugly moments. A few fights have erupted at Mains D'Or, which in French means "hands of gold," over something as petty as a crooked part; punches have been thrown and shirts ripped. "If a customer doesn't like the hairstyle, they might get a nasty attitude, jump out of the chair, and call you names," Fatima says, shaking her head in disbelief. "Instead of saying, 'Excuse me, miss, something is wrong with my hair.'

"But you try to satisfy them," she sighs. Sometimes she has to draw the line, though. Like when a sister arrives hours before an event requesting a rush job. The veteran braider refuses to hurry. "Why should I?" she asks, her dark brown pupils flashing. "So they can come back after the wedding and tell me that one of their braids fell out?"

The repetition of plaiting hair five days a week, nine hours a day, causes Fatima recurring neck, back, and joint pain. Still, customers sometimes complain when Fatima takes occasional breaks to catch her breath and rest her fingers, even if she's working a style that takes five or more hours to complete. What can make matters worse, she says, is that after she has toiled over teeny micro braids (about 150 to 200 per head), "Many New Yorkers don't tip." Out-of-state customers tend to be more generous. Clients from Connecticut, Philadelphia, Chicago, and even Ohio tend to tuck a few extra dollars in Fatima's palm. Tips are especially important at Mains D'Or, where employees fork out over 60 percent of their earnings to the owners.

Fatima's manner is gentle, accommodating. It is difficult to ruffle this quiet soul, but hurtful misconceptions about Africa upset her. Once, a customer asked if she had running water in her home in Africa. "Of course we do." Her voice arches unexpectedly. "People dis you, put you down. Like Africa don't have nothing. [In Africa] we own homes and have cars." What they don't have, she explains, is jobs. Fatima and Amadou both find that they fare better in America.

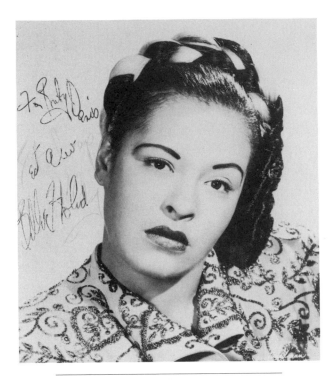

Lady Day branches beyond flower power, ca. 1941.

PHOTO: FRIEDMAN-ENGELER, SCHOMBERG
CENTER FOR RESEARCH IN BLACK CULTURE

But Amadou has settled into his adopted country faster than his wife. He actually enjoys the elbow-to-elbow hustle of big-city crowds; to him the code of the streets boils down to "respect." A few years ago, a would-be mugger tried to snatch Fatima's purse, but a neighbor stopped him. Afraid he would retaliate, Fatima didn't tell Amadou, but her neighbor did.

"Nobody messes with my family. I am no chicken, and I had to prove that to [the attacker] by kicking ass," Amadou proclaims in a rich baritone reminiscent of the singer Barry White.

Fatima still protests, but Amadou tells her, "I had to do something, or every time you came home, he would've tried to take your money."

A cloud of sadness comes over Fatima's face when I ask her if she has children. She does. All four live with her mother in Africa. My heart goes out to her. I don't have children yet, but I can imagine Fatima's pain. I doubt if I could be this strong. Trying to reunite her family is difficult. She's petitioned the U.S. embassy in Senegal, but they told her that she didn't make enough money to keep her children off welfare. So she travels to Senegal to see them. "Families are supposed to be together. All this time we're apart, on holidays and birthdays. . . . It hurts." Her voice trails off. "I know that someday we'll be together. It's what God decides."

• 1942 •

COOCHIE COO

Jimmy Rowles, a musician who played with Billie Holiday and often visited her dressing room, recalls that the singer was glamorous and uninhibited in an unusual way: "When I worked with her in 1942, she had her hair dyed red, and she had this dyed red [pubic hair] and she'd stand there with just a pair of shoes on, and I loved her all the more because she was so gorgeous, so beautiful."

—Donald Clarke, *Wishing on the Moon: The Life and Times of Billie Holiday*

I watch for a while longer as Fatima works, plaiting hair and burning ends, realizing that we aren't that different. We both want to be successful, healthy, loved, respected and understood. I say good-bye to her and wish her luck, and then head back downstairs en route to the subway on bustling 125th Street. All along the way I hear their soft voices: "Hair braiding, Miss?"

MADAM SPEAKS
Mark Richard Moss

Blond hair is a boon for black heads. All hail Mary J. Blige. And Tina Turner. Certainly the Supremes' abbreviated reunion tour would not have been complete without the obligatory blond wig. For a while, flaxen heads were sprouting up all over the place: Jada Pinkett Smith, Whitney Houston, Halle Berry, and, exemplifying the cross-generational aspect, the old warrior herself, poet Nikki Giovanni. Certainly she was not unaware of our black heritage because she helped to tell the story. . . .

While I'm not a gentleman who prefers blondes, I can't say I've totally discriminated against them. Once, four black women appeared at a mostly male gathering to watch a pay-per-view heavyweight fight. One stood out because of her dyed blond hair, but that's not why I

• 1969 •

GILDED BIRD

Maya Angelou's *I Know Why the Caged Bird Sings* is published. In this work, which will become a literary classic, Angelou recalls a youthful obsession: "Wouldn't they be surprised when one day I woke out of my black and ugly dream, and my real hair, which was long and blond, would take the place of the kinky mass that Momma wouldn't let me straighten?"

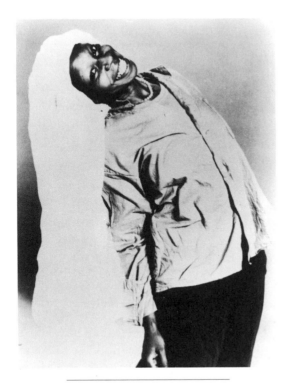

*Whoopi Goldberg acts out many a
black girl's fantasy.*

PHOTOFEST

ended up with her phone number. There were a couple of other attributes that quickened my pulse, which led to conversation and the promise of drinks at another time. Her hair color was of little concern because I wasn't planning to stick around that long. But as a product of the black consciousness movement, natural hair color was part of my litmus test in selecting a wife. I do wonder, though, where exactly should politically correct black people draw the hair color line?

I decided to ask a higher authority. And who better than Madam C. J. Walker? Yes, *that* Madam Walker, the mother of African-American beauty culture and a socially conscious race woman. Initially, I feared that she might not have kept current with the trends, having been out of the loop for eighty-one years. But I was elated to find just the opposite.

My interview took place in the tiny back room of an old house in Louisiana. The proprietor insisted that I keep information about the location on the "down low"; she works by appointment only and doesn't advertise. Discretion, she claims, minimizes encounters with "kooks."

As my host contacted the spirit world, Madam Walker materialized. I recognized her from her photographs: full-figured, no-nonsense, imposing. My intentions were to break the ice by summarizing the sixties and seventies, when "the struggle" was at full tilt. I wanted to give her a feel for how we went from "black is beautiful" to "blond is all that." But she stopped me. . . .

WALKER: That's enough, son. Let me explain something. I am in God's house, and from here we can see it all. I know everything that's happened since I got on the train.

MRM: Nice to know that the departed have more perks than what are commonly known.

WALKER: So how can I help you, honey?

MRM: As you know, a lot of black women have been dying their hair blond. Do you think they're going overboard in trying to beautify themselves?

WALKER: Son, you've got to see the big picture. When you look into the eyes of an African American, you see Africa. You see the Yoruba and the Fanti and the BaKonga tribes, to name just a few. You see their ceremonies and their villages and their clothes. These people have a passion for bright color.

MRM: So you're saying that the gold-top sisters of today are responding to archetypes from the ethnic collective unconscious?

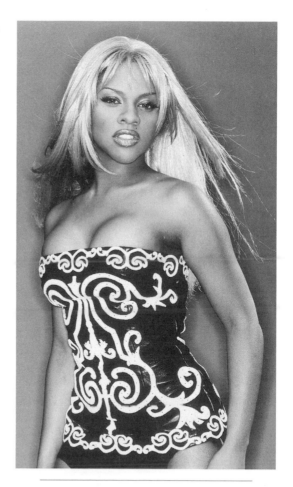

Lil' Kim, with the bluest eyes, and blondest hair money can buy, flaunts the fantasy.

PHOTOFEST/MARK BAPTISTE,
CORBIS OUTLINE

WALKER: What's that? I'm smart, honey, but I didn't go to Harvard.

MRM: What you're trying to say is that blacks' attraction to colors is in our roots?

WALKER: Yeah honey, didn't you ever hear about red being the Negro national color? Another thing, it's no secret that brown-skinned folks very often have red and gold undertones in their skin, which deep gold hair can set off pretty nicely.

MRM: During the late sixties, early seventies, I called myself radical. Had an Afro, a dashiki, and the whole nine. Then my father marries my third stepmother, a light-skinned younger woman with dyed blond hair. She turned out to be a decent stepmother. And she still dyes her hair, by the way.

WALKER: Why don't you ask her why the color?

MRM: I will. But I don't think I'll get an honest answer. She won't say, "I went blond because being redbone and blond during my heyday offered more opportunities than just being redbone." She won't be that honest.

WALKER: Her heyday was when? The fifties, sixties? Back then, only redbone colored women dared to go blond, and when they did, their excuse was, "My hair was cornflower yellow when I was a baby."

MRM: The cultural love of bright colors aside, do you think that bottle-blond black women are masquerading? The counterpart of Hillary Clinton in a big, bristling Afro wig?

WALKER: That's a good question. But there's no simple answer. You can look at black people with blond hair as getting a piece of the rock. It's a way of saying to white folks, I got what you got. But all that glitters ain't gold, honey, as any woman knows, who has over-processed her hair to the point where she's found it swirling down the drain.

MRM: *Vogue* magazine featured Lil' Kim and Mary J. Blige in a story about the two making the rounds during New York City's Fashion Week. The writer asked Lil' Kim's hairdresser, "How was her hair?" He says,

"Very blond. Very free. Very open. Very Ivana." Very Ivana—that bothers me.

WALKER: Yeah, who wants to be a bad imitation of something that's already fake? But then again, it's all illusion. That's why that makeup company hired those girls, because they're already outrageous and they can move a lot of lipstick. What's that other girl's name—Madonna? She up and did the same thing. It was like the second coming of Marilyn Monroe. Everybody's always scuffling around, trying to find some new way to look. For those girls, it's how they stay out of the unemployment line.

MRM: Have you heard that joke going around on the Internet?: "You know you're ghetto if you're a dark-skinned woman but you dye your hair blond because you think it makes you look lighter."

WALKER: If you're trying to do all that with a bottle of peroxide, you got more issues than what color your hair should be. How about you, Mark? What if you went home tonight and your wife had dyed her hair blond?

MRM: I'd say, Baby, I love you, but I'm not feeling that. One time she did come home with a streak of brown. It was cool, but blond is too flashy, too false. She might as well walk down Main Street in stiletto heels and a G-string.

WALKER: I don't know about all that, but some women do like the attention being blond brings. Tell you how much times have changed, in my day, women who wanted attention wore lipstick. We called it lip rouge, back then. You came out the house in that, it was considered pretty brazen.

MRM: That doesn't compare to Lil' Kim coming out on an awards show with one breast hanging out.

WALKER: No comparison at all. By the way, those sisters putting blond in their hair?

MRM: Yeah?

WALKER: Tell them to be careful. All those chemicals wreck our kind of hair. Folks call nappy hair "coarse" like it really is some kind of steel wool, but it's actually fragile and breaks off easy.

MRM: So it's the health of hair that concerns you most, not the symbolism?

WALKER: Always. I know what it's like to lose a head of hair. In my time, women weren't losing their hair because of dyes and perms, but on account of poor nutrition and bad scalp conditions. So when you ask me about what color people should *wear* their hair, that's not the main thing to ask. That's just the outside show. We got to deal with what's inside people's heads. Get that figured out and them blond questions will take care of themselves. People think I was trying to straighten everybody's head out. I was, but not with a hot comb. So tell me, did I answer your question?

MRM: More than you know.

WALKER: If you ever find yourself out this way, stop by and see me.

MRM: Thanks for the invitation. Forgive me if I say I hope it'll be a while.

WALKER: Forgiven.

• 2000 •

HEAD SCRATCHER

The two male announcers for NBC's broadcast of the French Open tennis tournament discuss Venus Williams' new hairstyle, but ultimately do not know what to say:

STAFF ANNOUNCER: What happened to the beads?

JOHN MCENROE: She's got some extra hair. Looks like some extensions, but . . .

Even two heads couldn't figure that one out, and McEnroe never finished the sentence.

Straight Talk

around 70 percent of black women in the United States—and an untold number of sisters in the diaspora—wear their hair straightened. Rejecting the notion that their black pride has paled, these sisters say, What's hair got to do with it? It's the advantages of straightened styles that they want, not the attributes of another race. In fact some women believe their fortunes are tied to their straightened tresses. Without a doubt, women like media mogul Oprah Winfrey and Congresswoman Maxine Waters have perfected an impeccably coiffed look that has helped them crack through a series of glass ceilings leading straight to the top.

IN OTHER WORDS . . .

"Good hair," a.k.a:
righteous grass
righteous moss

Hair historian Willie Morrow says that during slavery, moss that grew from trees was added to the hair for length, much as hair extensions are used today.

RELAX YOUR MIND!
Jenyne M. Raines

I am not ashamed to crow, I love my hair relaxed! Now, I didn't say that I am not also crying at any given moment about a problem that all of my armchair-dermatologist friends seem to believe stems from the chemical interaction, but that just goes with the territory. I love my relaxed hair—it's easy to groom, it bounces, it behaves, and for the most part it's a no-brainer! Although, with all of our newfound hair versatility—no hair; weaved-to-your-booty hanks; happily nappy locks—a permed head sounds, well, prehistoric. While we have wisely stored the conk and the blow-out kit on the dusty shelf of antiquity, I am telling you, relaxed hair accompanied this sister into the twenty-first century!

Of course, I have to ask myself why I am so gung-ho on a process that I know, on the basis of high school chemistry alone, is caustic. The active ingredient in your basic relaxer is sodium hydroxide—better known as lye—a substance that will break down another material, like the outer cuticle of your hair, upon contact, and ultimately destroy it. And then of course there is the no-lye lie. True, the "no-lye" relaxers don't contain sodium hydroxide as the active ingredient, but trust me, calcium hydroxide is just a milder form of lye. The key word is hydroxide! Now, I may have been dozing through the periodic-chart lesson, but the acid-oxide part I got.

What is the lure, a pull so strong that I, and so many other black women subject ourselves to a time-consuming, potentially balding process every eight weeks? *Gurrrrl, you don't know the half of it!*

As with everything else in life, the hair question always comes back to those three-hour evening phone calls with one of your sistafriends. You start with the general niceties, get in deep with the latest on your man-of-the-minute, or bemoan the fact that there is no man. Then your girl jumps in with her tired, boyfriend tirade or her "where-are-the-brothers?" wail. And we bring it all home with what? The old hair conversation. Now, if you thought the exchange on the brothers was animated, you ain't heard nothing until you hear my friends go on about their relaxed hair.

"I think my hair is falling out," says your pal.

"Really," you cluck sympathetically, although the last time you saw her, her flip was fly.

"Yeah," she sighs, "I am telling you, as soon as I get a husband, I am going to cut this stuff off and lock it up." Then you go through your bit about wanting to grow your perm out so that your hair can be healthier, but this new swingy layered cut seems to have the brothers hawking. Hmmm, in a not-so-subtle way, the conversation is back to men.

Oh, no, it can't be. Am I subjecting myself to sodium hydroxide on the regular for a date and, down the line, "that special brother" who gifts me with a Tiffany's ring box? Er, no, it can't be that deep, can it?

Now, I don't want to put anything else on the brothers—it's hard enough when you're seen as the personification of all things criminal or athletic and on top of that you can't catch a cab—but they do factor into the hair equation. Yes, according to the anthropologists, hair is a man thing because lush, long locks have signaled sexual attractiveness for men since caveman days. I'd just assumed that most brothers are mad for hair, the more of it the better being their general motto. I didn't know I had science backing me up. While most brothers are no longer duped by the long-hair-by-any-means-necessary tactics, they do insist on well-groomed tresses of any texture. Hence, my girls and I go to great lengths to keep men's heads turning. Of course, that doesn't explain why we're still home on Friday night. But that's our story, and we're sticking to it!

Why would anyone want to be a slave to a jar of chemicals or a smoking pressing comb? The nationalists among us insist it's because we're trying to look white, while the earthy crunchy contingent says we're not enlightened to our own beauty. "Our Kind of People" say it is the only way to go if you don't have blow-in-the-wind waves, and darling, make sure it's shoulder-length—at least! But the modern sister understands that this whole thing is about versatility, not Miss Ann.

I believe the relaxer's allure is in the ease it offers, and yes, it is informed by a bit of old-school thinking—a motivation that makes the rationale, "Well, broth-erman likes it," a lesser consideration.

Let's be brutally honest here. There is no ignoring the potentially devastating effects on the psyche when one falls short of what black folks consider the holy trinity: hair, skin color, and features. I don't have to kick the ballistics about the ideal "black" beauty. Whether she was yesterday's Cotton Club chorus girl or today's rap-video honey, she usually has long hair, café au lait skin, and delicate features. The rest of us were left to fight it out on the food chain by playing up whatever was closest to the ideal in any sector of the trinity. Being brown and the possessor of rounded features, the only thing I had "going for me" was soft hair that relaxed easily for a shoulder length, vaguely blow-in-the-wind sort of look. I ran with it.

Yes, this decision was made during my impressionable teen years in the sev-enties, and now that I am closer in age to receiving a social security check than a training bra, I realize that the old values of Negro Beauty 101 have been hard-wired into my brain.

Why, you ask, am I still holding on to and celebrating a look that for all intent and purpose was created in response to an idea as absurd and as antiquated as the Octoroon's Ball? I like it, damn it! True, the trinity is a rough concept to shake, but its dictatorial grip has loosened considerably. For me, my cocoa-colored complexion was always cool. I'll probably never be wild about my nose, but I've always loved my hair. And yes, I have done the Afro, Afro puffs, and cornrows, as well as the "grow the chemicals out" phase.

I have tried to grow my relaxed hair out several times. And I adored the crinkliness of the new growth, the cotton candy softness, and the beauty of it—until I had to put a comb through it. I would tell the stylist to do something with my hair but don't braid it, 'cause I don't look great with braids, and no curly Afro 'cause I haven't done that since seventh grade. Er, what was left? Yes, pull out the hot comb.

That's right, this doll has looked at life from both sides of the Afro pick, and at the end of a very long, follicularly challenged day, I still want straight hair. It's a matter of energy and my overall look and persona. And that is why my reasons to straighten aren't so complex and angst-ridden. Relaxed hair is part of how I see myself, and it is just as much a part of my identity as my curvy-heeled mules, short skirts, and laugh-a-lot personality.

Relaxed hair has evolved past the imitation of the white girl. It represents a lifelong bond and a ritual. And the straightening comb is a natural progression as Mom's three-braid special begins to look pretty juvenile. Mom puts the comb on the stove, breaks out the Sulfur 8, and pulls out the high chair; it becomes mother-daughter time. Straight hair signifies the passage to junior high school. For Dad, it is the beginning of the end of innocence. His little girl is growing up. Special occasions become that much more special because you are trundled off to the beauty parlor. My own hairdresser at fourteen! Is this how divas develop?

Going away to college means Mom relents for the relaxer. She won't be around to monitor the hair, and neither will Eula, the hairdresser, but the relaxer and the brouhaha that goes along with it help win new friends with conversations built on anecdotes, misinformation, and questions about who the best hairstylists are, what products make your hair grow, and omigod, it's touch-up time. You could reel the coldest sister into conversation if you had a kernel of info on how to keep that relaxed hair from breaking. To this day you can keep an exchange going between a woman from Tennessee and one from Togo with the basic question, What should I do with my relaxed hair?

The relaxer is also a factor in the dress-for-success formula. In corporate America or anywhere a suit and tie is de rigueur, so is straight, unobtrusive hair. As sisters started flooding the corporate gates, relaxed was the way to go. In fairness to whites, I never believed their endorsement of relaxed hair was because they thought we were trying to emulate them; it's just that it's less disturbing to their line of vision, and thus makes us a bit more palatable and easily rendered invisible. And really, it was conformity at its best. It's much easier to hold a sister back when her hair seems to have a strong point of view.

That's right; I am here to praise straightened hair, not to bury it in tired rhetoric about wanting to be white. Really, that concept is so 1969. A more radical concept that doesn't get much play is the reality that relaxed hair is about power and profits. Relaxed hair is the cornerstone of the $1.7 billion we spend on hair each year. The first black person to earn a million dollars, Madam C. J. Walker, made her fortune in hair salves. Then George Johnson perfected the relaxer and gave us Ultra Sheen's no-base creme relaxer. Hairstylists profited because more than any other style, the relaxer meant repeat business.

Folks, it gets deep. Before the white companies got involved or wanted anything to do with us (just yesterday), you had a whole second tier of distributors—middlemen, really—who got the product from the company salesman to the hairstylist. Come on, let's do the math. The desire for straight hair that lasts for more than a week begets the relaxer. The relaxer begets, if done properly, the hairstylist. The stylist begets an arsenal of ancillary cleansing and conditioning products. You go home with a line of hair products to add to the arsenal of grooming utensils. Your new bouncy 'do begets a minimum of three styling products—moisturizer (Note: grease is old-school), sheen spray, and holding spray. And two weeks begets another trip to the stylist, or—for the penny pinchers—every eight weeks to start the cycle again.

Kaching!

For the longest time, relaxed hair, like hip-hop, was a black thing, a product we created, somewhat controlled, and prospered from. Now, just as with hip-hop, we've lost our grip, and the profits are being siphoned out of the community.

Relaxed hair also signifies power of another sort: the power of choice. When your hair is relaxed properly—I am not talking about over-processed limp, broken hair—you can have fun. Scrunch up your freshly washed hair with styling gel and let it air-dry, and you have ringlets. Blow-dry it smooth and let it hang for black girl *au naturel.* Blow and curl for a finished look. Catch it up in barrettes. Swoop it up in a topknot. Headband it for a black Muffy look. Twist it, braid it, tuck it into a neat chignon. All of these 'dos can be done with ease until touch-up time, which is akin to Cinderella's coach turning into a pumpkin.

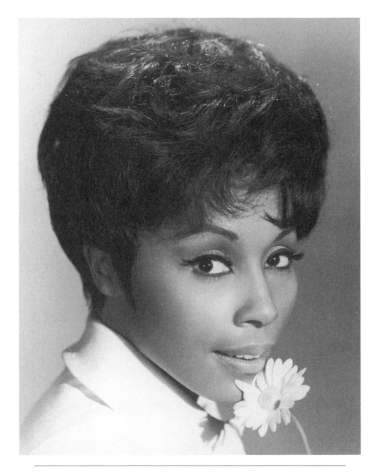

In 1968, Diahann Carroll, as "Julia," was the first black woman to star in a network TV series. Her sophisticated cut showed how far the press & curl had come since the 1950s.

PHOTOFEST

I love my relaxed hair. I can't imagine myself without it. And while theories may abound about why I and the other 70 percent or so of my sisters sport relaxed hair, the reason is ultimately one of freedom. My choice is tempered with self-understanding and a healthy dose of self-love. The tale of my mane is a love story—a story of bonding, burning, wishing, hoping, frying, dyeing, and ultimately, of accepting who I am and having the bravura to go for it. No, it's not about the brothers. And it was never about the white girls. (And when you really look beyond the white-girl hype, you'll see they're struggling with their hair, too.) It's not just a black thing. And really, who cares? It's all about me . . . mostly old-school bobbed, sometimes shagged, but always relaxed and laughing!

SISTER SANCTUARY

Mama Nettie's House of Beauty was a gathering place for women. A sanctuary. For it was in her parlor that women unsnapped their girdled souls, unclinched their fists and relaxed the lines in their foreheads. They were free at Mama Nettie's. There, in the midst of the sweet smell of Royal Crown or Dixie Peach, heated with a straightening comb or a curling iron, and the musk of bodies worn by a week's work, the women's laughter had the rhythm of a revival song.

—Angelene Jamison Hall, novel in progress

THE OTHER MOTHER OF BLACK BEAUTY CULTURE

Though she was running neck and neck with Madam C. J. Walker to re-dress the heads of black women with her Wonderful Hair Grower, history has not remembered Annie Malone as well as the Madam. Beginning her training in the fields with an old black woman herb doctor and continuing it in a high school chemistry course, Malone in 1900 began to

▪ 1918 ▪

During a concert tour, the "celebrated Negro tenor" Roland Hayes visited Poro College in St. Louis with his mother, a simple, deeply religious woman from rural Georgia. In a memoir, he recalled that the "proprietress [Annie Malone] had accumulated quite a comfortable fortune from ointments which made kinky hair straight. . . . Ma walked about amongst the laboratories and classrooms quoting Ecclesiastes on the subject of vanity."

manufacture her hair formula in a house she rented for $5 a month in Lovejoy, Illinois. She and her sister went door to door, selling the special concoction. Later she opened Poro College in St. Louis to train agents in her Poro Beauty System, and was a philanthropist and community leader.

IN OTHER WORDS . . .

CONK: Derivation of "congollene," the term black men gave to a mixture of sodium hydroxide (lye) and starch, applied to the head to remove the kink from tightly curled hair. In the 1930s, '40s, and '50s, the style was popular among black male entertainers, boxers, and hustlers.

KINK-OUT: General term for any type of hair straightener.

WHEN BLACK HAIR TANGLES
WITH WHITE POWER
Mariame Kaba

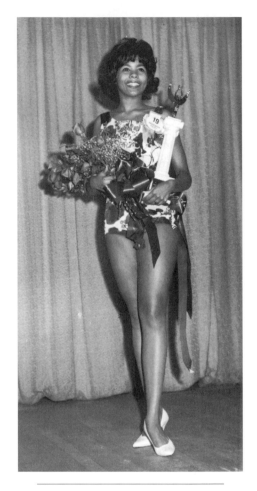

Described in a 1964 newspaper as a "lovely Negro lass," this beauty pageant contestant was a winner with her thick flip.

CORBIS/BETTMAN UPI

A free black man named Hodges gave a public demonstration of a "hair kink straightener" to a group of blacks at a hall in New York City in 1856. According to a *New York Times* report of the event, Hodges selected a man with a head full of nappy hair and paid him to be his subject. Slowly and methodically, Hodges combed the secret mixture through the man's head, telling the crowd of the potion's miraculous powers as the hair gradually became straight.

Everything seemed to be going swimmingly when the demonstration was interrupted by a woman who pushed her way to the front of the crowd, screaming her objections to the process.

"If blacks were meant to have straight hair," she shouted, "God would have given it to them."

A few people in the crowd yelled out for her to be quiet, but she would not. Then a fight broke out. Hodges rushed over to calm the brawling spectators, but when he returned to his demonstration and resumed combing his volunteer's hair, clumps began to hit the floor. In the end, the volunteer was half bald. Under the pretense of getting something from the other room, Hodges excused himself, and that was the last anybody saw of him.

Today the practice of hair straightening has become commonplace. Though a process that often requires many hours and much expense, roughly three-quarters of black women consider the time and financial investment worth it, according to Kathy Russell, coauthor of *The Color Complex: The Politics of Skin Color Among African Americans.* Why do so many black women submit to this sometimes painful practice? My research suggests that it is not a reflection of what I call "white power envy." Black women "take the heat" to achieve access to the economic and social resources within American society. (Of course, there are other powerful incentives for straightening one's hair, which

The Kitchen, *1997 (acrylic on board).*

DANIEL MINTER

have more to do with gaining social acceptance from family, friends, and men. And these usually result from pressures *within* the community—but that's not my focus here.)

Before I explore the interplay between black women's heads and society, let me step back a moment to discuss one theory, which holds that a woman who straightens her hair has a poor self-image. Some analysts build their entire theory on this one notion. They point to the straightening of hair, the bleaching of skin, and the preference for things "white" or "light" as proof. They go on to assert that these choices are attributable to the influences of the dominant white American society, in which black skin is defined as inferior. The antidote, these analysts suggest, is that blacks embrace "natural" or "African" hairstyles to uplift their self-image and cure pathological tendencies.

I call this interpretation of black behavior "the social pathology model." Some of its proponents maintain that blacks must rediscover their "natural" beauty in order to free themselves of self-hate. If they embrace their "African" features (broad nose, thick lips, dark skin, nappy hair), the theory holds, they will negate the white beauty aesthetic that is force-fed to them on a daily basis. These critics have argued for embracing African consciousness and style. While their notions may hold some validity, I find them to be lacking. My research suggests that, if indeed black women are adopting the "white standard of beauty," it's usually only as a means to an end.

Anita,* a 32-year-old housing specialist, offers this insight: "I wear my hair straight so that I can fit in. My mother said that if I didn't have 'good hair,' I would have no hope of getting a job, a husband, or any real respect in society."

I've heard this reasoning from a number of women whose experience challenges the social-pathology model. They place the source of the "problem" in the demands of society rather than in the "psychological" realm. While devalued black features can indeed lead to an "inferiority complex," I think that most black women who straighten their hair are not suffering from one. Rather they seek access to the resources that have been traditionally reserved for white men and women in this country. Black women are in search of some of the privileges that

---

*I have changed the names of my informants to protect their anonymity.

the "dominant" culture enjoys—a piece of the pie. And in the United States, where white men continue to control the institutions of consequence, they rightly associate whiteness with power.

African Americans have good reason to believe that a "white-like" appearance is a key determinant in economic success and social advancement. In *Black Women in America,* editor Darlene Clark Hine suggests that historically, "Black women with lighter skin and straighter hair gained higher paying jobs in the labor market and fared better socially, especially in marriages to wealthier Black men, who tended to choose women with those characteristics."

Since slavery, whites have rewarded blacks for looking almost white: "People with African ancestry and light skin have long known a relative advantage in American society," journalist Keith Woods writes in an article titled "Shades of Racism." E. Franklin Frazier makes a similar argument in his landmark 1957 study *Black Bourgeoisie,* in which he points out that as offspring of white slave-masters, light-skinned blacks were often spared from backbreaking fieldwork and from the overseer's whip. They usually served as house slaves where they enjoyed a better living standard than their darker-skinned counterparts. At night, they often laid their curly heads to rest in the "Big House," and in the morning they might don the master's and mistress's nicer hand-me-downs, sometimes wearing them during a reading or writing lesson. In the end, these light-skinned slaves were more likely to be freed by their masters. And when the Civil War ended, Frazier goes on to say, light-skinned families maintained their status, forming the top of black America's class structure.

A number of social scientists have explored the relationship between skin color and hair texture in black social and economic advancement. Verna Keith and Cedric Herring's research published in 1991 showed that skin tone and other such traits were more strongly related to one's class ranking than things like one's parent's socioeconomic status. A few years earlier, bell hooks wrote of a discussion about the importance of wearing hair straight for job interviews with students at Spelman College. Hooks observed that the women were "convinced, and probably rightly so, that their chances of finding good jobs would be enhanced if they had straight hair."

Clearly, African-American women are aware that Caucasian-like features are conducive to success in this society. As long as this is the case, I expect that black women will continue to straighten their hair in pursuit not of whiteness but of white power. The authors of *The Color Complex* echo this view when they write, "For African Americans embracing whiteness is a matter of economic, social, and political survival."

Some of the proponents of the social pathology model are content to simply attribute the practice of hair straightening to racism. This is without a doubt part of the answer. However, that group often ignores or misses the complicated interplay between racism, classism, and sexism. Their analysis suggests that race tends to take precedence over other aspects of social relations, such as gender and class. Race does provide the framework through which we conceive of some hair as "good" and other hair as "bad." However, hair becomes a more complex topic for black women because they are women and also because they are in an economically precarious position in the American social structure. It's obvious that gender plays an important role in this, since black men don't feel the same need to straighten their hair. Neither does the majority culture, which places additional pressure on black women by being unwilling to accept some black hairstyles.

This resistance is embedded in a clash between a black beauty aesthetic and traditional business norms. Dress codes and rules governing proper office attire are long-standing and often go unchallenged. The emphasis is on presenting a "professional" look. For years many women in black America have complained that when they wear their hair "naturally," they conflict with their supervisors. Others have complained that wearing natural styles has negatively influenced their chances of getting a job in the first place. Thus straightened hair became the norm and commonly accepted as proper grooming etiquette.

When news reporter Dorothy Reed of KGO-TV came to work one day in 1980 wearing cornrows, the station suspended her, contending that her hairdo was not consistent with an image that they wanted to promote. Many black journalists came to her defense, taking issue with her employer. Cries of discrimination and racism rang out, and in 1981 Reed was reinstated to her position. But that was the same year that Renee Rogers sued American Airlines over her right to wear braids on the job, and lost her case. That furor soon died down, only to be resurrected five years later with much stronger resistance from black women in other walks of life.

The tug-of-war continued when, in 1986, Cheryl Tatum, a restaurant cashier at a Hyatt hotel in Washington, D.C., was approached by her personnel director and asked to "unbraid her hair" because the chain "barred extreme and unusual hair styles," according to a 1987 article in the *New York Daily News* by E. R. Shipp.

Tatum refused the order, she said, so she was forced to resign. Tatum and three other Washington area women then filed complaints against the Hyatt with the federal Equal Employment Opportunity Commission. A year later Hyatt amended its policy to state that: "After careful consideration of several requests made by our employees, the executive committee has reviewed our grooming policy and has revised our hair policy. Hairstyles must not be extreme or unusual and should be appropriate for the health, safety and grooming standards of your department and the hotel. Multi-braided hair, a current acceptable fashion among women is permitted as long as it is well-groomed and neat."

In 1987 Pamela Mitchell, a part-time reservationist at the J. W. Marriott Hotel, decided she was more committed to her freedom than to her job. When told that her cornrows were inappropriate and "too extreme," she decided to keep the style and quit the company.

"I see it as an expression of culture, and the principle involved here is more important than my job," Mitchell explained. The same battles continued into the 1990s with complaints being lodged against a number of companies including Hertz, Wendy's and American Airlines (once again). In most of these cases, the companies amended their dress codes but the complainants received no settlements. One notable exception is Pamela Mitchell who settled her case with Marriott for $40,000 which also agreed to pay an additional amount of $15,000 in legal fees.

Many people argue that what lies at the heart of these objections and policies are racism and intolerance. They see the fight as an attempt to make black women conform to white standards. Others view it simply as a form of control and of "putting black women in their place." Many black woman simply opt for straight styles to avoid being singled out for punishment.

"I have to do it to look presentable and professional," Laura, a thirty-year-old attorney, told me. "If a lawyer wears braids, an Afro, or dreads, I think that she is even more disadvantaged than just being black and a woman. I don't want to draw more attention to myself."

Ultimately, for many, the choice becomes simple. One dean of students at Spelman College reportedly told her students that each "has to decide what's more important: the way she wears her hair or the position she is currently seeking."

In this context, then, a hairstyle is chosen to escape social and economic disadvantage. The economically vulnerable position that many black women find themselves in dissuades them from rocking the boat. But in striving for "white" power, they pour millions of dollars into hair products and treatments that cause an economic drain on their limited resources. Still, many see the investment as worth it.

So while powerful incentives within and without the black community help shape cultural practices, it is logical, not pathological, for black women to straighten their hair in America. Understood in this context, hair straightening can be viewed as an adaptive strategy. And while it is likely that a number of our ancestors could have indeed suffered from low self-esteem, and might even have straightened their hair in a desperate attempt to imitate white appearance, motives—like people—change over time.

Through my interviews, I found that black women's search for love, attention, and access to economic resources has in some way become tangled up with their hair issues, which makes me reflect on a few wise words from journalist Kristal Brent Zook: "The meaning of hair for Black women remains complicated. To me, Black nationalists who wear their kinks as badges of authenticity, judging at every turn, are just as dangerous as processed beauty queens. The constant weight of our hair, making us more or less Black, or special depending on the day, the weather and the style of our 'dos—is so heavy. How much longer must we shoulder the burden of having it represent all that we are?"

HOT COMB
Natasha Trethewey

Halfway through an afternoon
of coca cola bottles sweating rings
on veneered tabletops and the steel drone
of window fans above the silence

in each darkened room, I open a stiff drawer
and find the old hot combs, black
with grease, the teeth still pungent
as burning hair. One is small, fine-toothed
as if for a child. Holding it,
I think of my mother's slender wrist,
the curve of her neck as she leaned over
the stove, her eyes shut as she pulled
the wooden handle and laid flat the wisps
at her temples. The heat in our kitchen
made her glow that morning I watched her
wincing, the hot comb singeing her brow,
sweat glistening above her lips,
her face made strangely beautiful
as only suffering can do.

IN OTHER WORDS . . .

GREASE: The déclassé term that refers to hair preparations with a petroleum or beeswax base. The almighty lubricator, a jar of blue grease, was as much of a staple in the black household as the oil painting of Jesus, Martin Luther King, and John F. Kennedy. Ironically, the thick pomade does not eradicate dryness, but it did make for some entertaining commercials. Who can forget that paean to black pride from Afro Sheen: "Watu wazuri, use Afro Sheen . . . beautiful people use Afro Sheen."

A SLICK HISTORY OF HAIR GREASE

From palm oil and shea butter to:

hog lard
chicken fat
Dax

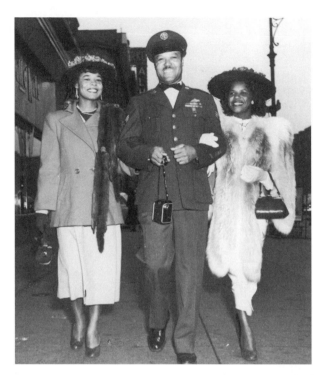

Nu Nile
Brilliantine
Royal Crown
Dixie Peach
Apex
Sulfur 8
Alberto VO5
Vitapoint
Posner Bergamot
Lustrasilk
Ultra Sheen
Hot Six Oil
jojoba
carrot oil

UPI-CORBIS/BETTMAN

*Whether it's 1952 in Harlem, or
1996 in Beaufort, South Carolina,
Easter is a big hair day.*

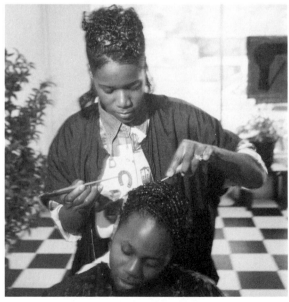

JULES T. ALLEN/CORBIS

STRAIGHTENING OUR HAIR
bell hooks

On Saturday mornings we would gather in the kitchen to get our hair fixed—that is, straightened. Smells of burning grease and hair, mingled with the scent of our freshly washed bodies, with collard greens cooking on the stove, with fried fish. We did not go to the hairdressers. Mamma fixed our hair. Six daughters—there was no way we could have afforded hairdressers. In those days, this process of straightening black women's hair with a hot comb was not connected in my mind with the effort to look white, to live out standards of beauty set by white supremacy. It was connected solely with rites of initiation into womanhood. To arrive at that point where one's hair could be straightened was to move from being perceived as child (whose hair could be neatly combed and braided) to being almost a woman. It was this moment of transition my sisters and I longed for.

Hair pressing was a ritual of black women's culture—of intimacy. It was an exclusive moment when black women (even those who did not know one another well) might meet at home or in the beauty parlor to talk with one another, to listen to the talk. It was as important a world as that of the male barbershop—mysterious, secret. It was a world where the images constructed as barriers between one's self and the world were briefly let go, before they were made again. It was a moment of creativity, a moment of change.

I wanted this change even though I had been told all my life that I was one of the "lucky" ones, because I had been born with "good hair"—hair that was

• 1988 •

Director Spike Lee spoofs the straight versus nappy debate in *School Daze*. In "Madame Re-Re's Beauty Salon," the mostly light-skinned, long-haired "wannabes" battle it out with the mostly dark-skinned, short-haired "jigaboos."

fine, almost straight—not good enough, but still good. Hair that had no nappy edges, no "kitchen," that area close to the neck that the hot comb could not reach. This "good hair" meant nothing to me when it stood as a barrier to my entering this secret black woman world. I was overjoyed when Mama finally agreed that I could join the Saturday ritual, no longer looking on but patiently waiting my turn. I have written of this ritual: "For each of us getting our hair pressed is an important ritual. It is not a sign of our longing to be white. There are no white people in our intimate world. It is a sign of our desire to be women. It is a gesture that says we are approaching womanhood." Before we reach the appropriate age we wear braids, plaits that are symbols of our innocence, our youth, our childhood. Then, we are comforted by the parting hands that comb and braid, comforted by the intimacy and bliss. There is a deeper intimacy in the kitchen on Saturdays when hair is pressed, when fish is fried, when sodas are passed around, when soul music drifts over the talk. It is a time without men. It is a time when we work as women to meet each other's needs, to make each other feel good inside, a time of laughter and outrageous talk.

Since the world we lived in was racially segregated, it was easy to overlook the relationship between white supremacy and our obsession with hair. Even though black women with straight hair were perceived to be more beautiful than those with thick, fuzzy hair, it was not overtly related to a notion that white women were a more appealing female group or that their straight hair set a beauty standard black women were struggling to live out. While this was probably the ideological framework from which the process of straightening black women's hair emerged, it was expanded so that it became a real space of black women bonding through ritualized, shared experience. The beauty parlor was a space of consciousness raising, a space where black women shared life stories—hardships, trials, gossip; a place where one could be comforted and one's spirit renewed. It was for some women a place of rest where one did not need to meet the demands of children or men. It was the one hour some folk would spend "off their feet," a soothing, restful time of meditation and silence. These positive empowering implications of the ritual of pressing mediate but do not change negative implications. They exist alongside all that is negative.

Within white supremacist capitalist patriarchy, the social and political context in which the custom of black folks straightening our hair emerges, it represents an imitation of the dominant white group's appearance and often indicates internalized racism, self-hatred, and/or low self-esteem. During the 1960s black people who actively worked to critique, challenge, and change white racism pointed to the way in which black people's obsession with straight hair reflected a colonized mentality. It was at this time that the natural hairdo, the Afro, became fashionable as a sign of cultural resistance to racist oppression and as a celebration of blackness. Naturals were equated with political militancy. Many young black folks found just how much political value was placed on straightened hair as a sign of respectability and conformity to social expectations when they ceased to straighten their hair. When black liberation struggles did not lead to revolutionary change in society, the focus on the political relationship between appearance and complicity with white racism ceased, and folks who once sported Afros began to straighten their hair.

In keeping with the move to suppress black consciousness and efforts to be self-defining, white corporations began to acknowledge black people and most especially black women as potential consumers of products they could provide, including hair-care products. Permanents especially designed for black women eliminated the need of pressing and the hot comb. They not only cost more but also took much of the economy and profit out of black communities, out of the pockets of black women who had previously reaped the material benefits (see Manning Marable's *How Capitalism Underdeveloped Black America* [South End Press 1985]). Gone was the context of ritual, of black women bonding. Seated under noisy hair dryers, black women lost a space for dialogue, for creative talk.

Stripped of the positive bonding rituals that traditionally surrounded the experience, black women straightening our hair seemed more and more to be exclusively a signifier of white supremacist oppression and exploitation. It was clearly a process that was about black women changing their appearance to imitate white people's looks. This need to look as much like white people as possible, to look safe, is related to a desire to succeed in a white world. Before desegregation black people could worry less about what white folks thought about their hair. In a discussion about beauty at Spelman College, students talked about the importance of wearing straight hair when seeking jobs. They were convinced, and probably rightly so, that their chances of finding good jobs would be enhanced if they had straight hair. When asked to elaborate, they focused on the connection between radical politics and natural hairdos, whether short or braided. One woman wearing a short natural told of purchasing a straight wig for her job search. No one in the discussion felt they were free to wear their hair in natural styles without reflecting on the possible negative consequences. Often older black adults, especially parents, respond quite negatively to natural hairdos. I shared with the group that when I arrived home with my hair in braids shortly after accepting my job at Yale, my parents told me I looked disgusting.

Despite many changes in racial politics, black women continue to obsess about their hair, and straightening hair continues to be serious business. It continues to tap into the insecurity black women feel about our value in this white supremacist society. When I talk with groups of women at various college campuses and with black women in our communities, there seems to be a consensus that our obsession with hair in general reflects continued struggles with self-esteem and self-actualization. We talk about the extent to which black women perceive our hair as the enemy, as a problem we must solve, a territory we must conquer. Above all it is a part of our black female body that must be controlled. Most of us were not raised in environments where we learned to regard our hair as sensual or beautiful in an unprocessed state. Many of us talk about situations where white people ask to touch our hair when it is unprocessed, then show surprise that the texture is soft or feels good. In the eyes of many white folks and other nonblack folks, the natural Afro looks like steel wool or a helmet. Responses to natural hairstyles worn by black women usually reveal the extent to which our natural hair is perceived in white supremacist culture as not only ugly but frightening. We also internalize that fear. The extent to which we are comfortable with our hair usually reflects on our overall feelings about our bodies.

In numerous discussions with black women about hair, I have found that one of the strongest factors preventing them from wearing unprocessed hairstyles is the fear of losing other people's approval and regard. Heterosexual black women talk about the extent to which black men respond more favorably to women with straight or straightened hair. Lesbian women point to the fact that many of them do not straighten their hair, raising the question of whether or not this gesture is fundamentally linked to heterosexism and a longing for male approval.

When my black women students read about race and physical beauty, they are reminded of periods in childhood when they were overcome with longing for straight hair, as it was so associated with desirability, with being loved. Few women had received affirmation from family, friends, or lovers when choosing not to straighten their hair, and many tell stories about receiving advice from everyone, including total strangers, urging them to understand how much more attractive they would be if they would fix (straighten) their hair. When I interviewed for my job at Yale, white female advisers who had never before commented on my hair encouraged me not to wear braids or a large natural to the interview. Although they did not say straighten your hair, they were suggesting that I change my hairstyle so that it would most resemble theirs, so that it would indicate a certain conformity. I wore braids, and no one seemed to notice. When I was offered the job, I did not ask if it mattered whether or not I wore braids. I tell this story to my students so that they will know by this one experience that we do not always need to surrender our power to be self-defining to succeed in an endeavor. Yet I have found that the issue of hairstyle comes up again and again with students when I give lectures. At one conference on black women and leadership I walked into a packed auditorium, my hair unprocessed, and all over the place. The vast majority of black women seated there had straightened hair. Many of them looked at me with hostile, contemptuous stares. I felt as though I was being judged on the spot as someone out on the fringe, an undesirable.

A number of black women have argued that straightened hair is not necessarily a signifier of low self-esteem. They argue that it is a survival strategy; it is easier to function in this society with straightened hair. There are fewer hassles. Or, as some folk stated, straightened hair is easier to manage, takes less time.

Individual preferences (whether rooted in self-hate or not) cannot negate the reality that our collective obsession with hair straightening reflects the psychology of oppression and the impact of racist colonization. Together racism and sexism daily reinforce to all black females via the media and mass culture that we will not be considered beautiful or desirable if we do not change ourselves, especially our hair. We cannot resist this socialization if we deny that white supremacy informs our efforts to construct self and identity.

Without organized struggles like the ones that happened in the 1960s and early 1970s, individual black women must struggle alone to acquire the critical consciousness that would enable us to examine issues of race and beauty, our personal choices, from a political standpoint. There are times when I think of straightening my hair just to change my style, just for fun. Then I remind myself that even though such a gesture could be simply playful on my part, an individual expression of desire, I know that such a gesture would carry other implications beyond my control. The reality is: straightened hair is linked historically and currently to a system of racial domination that impresses upon black people, and especially black women, that we are not acceptable as we are, that we are not beautiful. To make such a gesture as an expression of individual freedom and choice would make me complicit with a politic or domination that hurts us. It is easy to surrender this freedom. It is more important that black women resist racism and sexism in every way; that every aspect of our self-representation be a fierce resistance, a radical celebration of our care and respect for ourselves.

Even though I have not had straightened hair for a long time, this has not meant that I am able to really enjoy or appreciate my hair in its natural state. For years I still considered it a problem—it wasn't naturally nappy enough to make a decent interesting Afro; it was too thin. These complaints expressed my continued dissatisfaction. True liberation of my hair came when I stopped trying to control it in any state and just accepted it as it is. It has been only in recent years that I have ceased to worry about what other people say about my hair. Only in recent years have I felt consistent pleasure in washing, combing, and caring for my hair. These feelings remind me of the pleasure and comfort I felt as a child sitting between my mother's legs, feeling the warmth of her body and being as she combed and braided my hair. In a culture of domination, one that is essentially anti-intimacy, we must struggle daily to remain in touch with ourselves and our bodies, with one another. This is especially true for black women and men, as it is our bodies that have been so often devalued, burdened, wounded in alienated labor. Celebrating our bodies, we participate in a liberatory struggle that frees mind and heart.

A RIO CRIME

Laura Sullivan

ANDRE: Let me ask you a question: Are you chemically free?
AUDIENCE: No. [softly]

ANDRE: Do you wanna be?
AUDIENCE: Yes! [loudly]

ANDRE: Let me hear you say that word—
AUDIENCE: Rio!

ANDRE: Say it again!
AUDIENCE: Rio!

ANDRE: Say it again!
AUDIENCE: Rio!

—Dialogue from the Rio Hair Naturalizer infomercial

The introduction of a product called the Rio Hair Naturalizer in the early 1990s marked a particularly provocative and frightening moment in the history of black women's hair care. Shown in 1993 and 1994 on late-night TV, the infomercial featured black people sitting around tables in a comedy-club-like atmosphere, seemingly enjoying themselves as emcee Andre Desmond, a hairdresser, along with his cohost Mary, promised them "freedom" from nappy hair. Like all infomercials, the one for Rio blurred the line between TV programming and TV commercials. But people bought the concept, and sales of the product took off and remained brisk—until the lawsuits started rolling in

Rio gained credibility, in part, by tapping one of the most persuasive elements of the civil rights movement: its religious tone. Yet unlike earlier black liberation efforts, Rio had nothing to do with political or economic parity. It spoke, instead, to the right of black women to be able to shake their hair like white women. In the infomercial, Andre sounds like a preacher when he declares that one of the volunteers from the audience will be transformed to have the same smooth, bouncy hair that his cohost Mary enjoys: "When she comes back, she too shall move her hair, and it shall look and feel like Mary's," Andre proclaims. The use of the biblical-sounding "shall," as well as the biblical name Mary, suggests an edict by a religious leader, or even by God himself.

Mimicking the call-and-response tradition of the black church, Andre continuously asks the audience to yell "Rio!" and to "Say it again." This tactic serves to uplift the product to the level of savior, and equates salvation with having hair that can be straightened without use of lye. In the following exchange, Mary makes the religious link even more overt:

MARY: You want to become chemically free?
WOMAN: Yes.

MARY: Can we hear an "Amen" for that?
WOMAN: Amen.

MARY: She's gonna become chemically free here!
AUDIENCE: [cheers, claps]

The suggestion of conversion is even more explicit when Mary tries to convince audience members that they need the chemical freedom (read: salvation) that Rio offers:

MARY: You're going to feel my hair, you're going to see it, and by the time you leave here today [she points around the audience], I'm going to convert every single one of you, because you are going to be chemically free—okay?

The conversion is complete when audience volunteers reappear after being "transformed" by the product. Mary heralds the event: "And now, the moment you've been waiting for—the miracle moment of Rio. . . . I am about to bring out Andre with his three ladies."

In the infomercial, "good" hair is associated with the characteristics of "white" hair: straight, bouncy, touchable, manageable. Mary continuously shakes her hair throughout the "show," and the audience responds with awe. "Bad" hair, on the other hand, is kinky, unshakable, and rough to the touch, traits generally associated with black hair. The infomercial repeatedly reminds viewers that they should avoid bad hair, which also includes damaged, chemically treated hair.

Rio's marketing campaign went over big. Roughly 340,000 people purchased the product, according to court documents. Sadly, in the process, the "salvation" it promised played upon the anxieties many black women feel as a result of living in a racist and sexist culture. Still, the concept of making themselves more alluring resounded for many black women, even as they may have recognized the oppressiveness in the message.

AROUSING MALE DESIRE

The Rio infomercial suggests that the primary goal for black women is to receive approval and affection from men:

ANDRE: [to male audience members]: How many women have you seen walking up and down the streets that you want to walk up and touch their hair? And now, how many people have you seen that you say, "I'd rather not touch that"?

AUDIENCE: Oooh . . .

ANDRE: [to the women]: Men like to play in your hair. And I'm going to first tell you the warning— You start using [Rio], and you start living the life of a real girl, and your hair gets to this stage— [To Mary] Shake your hair again, Mary. [She does] You . . . run the risk of men coming up and saying things to you, like, "How you doing?" or "Can we do this?" or "Can we do that?"

MARY [to Andre]: Hi, baby!

[Andre puts his arm around her]

AUDIENCE: Whooo . . . [hoots, hollers]

ANDRE: Again, it's the world's first all-natural, gradual naturalizer. Each time you use Rio, you come away with softer, more manageable hair. This is your answer. [Looks into the camera, presumably at the viewer at home.] And if you're watching, call that number, because this truly is the answer. [A phone number appears at the bottom of the screen.]

If Rio Hair was "the answer," what was the problem? On one level, it was racism itself, and Mary's shakeable hair became a symbol for the "freedom" sought by black people in America. Rather than rendering blackness acceptable, it called for women to cease to "mark" themselves as people of color. To become what Andre called "a real girl," attract a man, and hold on to him, a black woman had to adhere to rigid standards based upon the characteristics of white women.

As a white woman, this disturbs me. I don't enjoy being the object of the dominant culture's definition of beauty. It hurts all us women, and makes me the

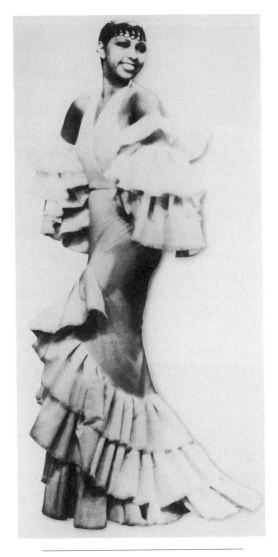

Noted for her many dazzling hair incarnations, in a career that spanned more than fifty years, Josephine Baker was initially considered too young, thin and dark for stardom. "What a wonderful revenge for an ugly duckling," she once said of her fame.

PHOTOFEST

object of many black women's resentment. In this and other ways, Western culture insidiously keeps us powerless by keeping us women separate from one another, so we don't build coalitions across race lines. Instead we are positioned to see each other as enemies, or as potential competitors in the quest to snag a "good man."

My desire to understand the realities of black women's hair care stems not from some voyeuristic position of privilege and judgment, but rather from the recognition that learning about people in identity positions different from our own, and seeing how the oppression of that group functions, are crucial steps for those of us positioned on the oppressor end of the spectrum. That way we may have the awareness to stop participating in that oppression as much as possible, and to work in tandem with other groups to end it.

MEN ON TOP

Andre repeatedly asks Mary to "do it again," and she obeys, shaking her hair for the audience. Throughout the video, he commands several women to shake their heads, and in fact the video ends as he instructs the volunteers and Mary, "Shake your heads, again, ladies," and the women all vigorously shake their heads—lowered, of course—while the audience claps and cheers loudly.

Andre's role in the infomercial indicates that even with its reliance on feminist rhetoric—highlighting the control and power afforded women by the product—males are still the ultimate arbiters of beauty standards. One audience volunteer in the infomercial explains why she's so happy with her new look: "When I walked in the room, my boyfriend didn't know who I was. He was like, 'Is that Jocia?' I had to tell him; he was excited."

I am at my apartment complex pool playing with some of my young friends; they are black children aged six to thirteen. Kareem, the oldest, says to me, "Laura, you have good hair!" I'm startled. "It's so soft and so silky," he continues, and then comes up and touches it. He sounds just like the man in the infomercial. I want to say that I think Jasmine, who is eight, and Janae, who is six, whose tight tresses are fashioned into braids, also have good hair, but I'm afraid he'll contradict me. The girls just look at me as if to say: The male has made his pronouncement. I feel powerless, with mere words, to convince them otherwise.

UGLY WAYS

As one e-mailer to an online chat site that I used to frequent noted, "many black women have had traumatic emotional experiences while getting their hair done. Writer Lisa Jones describes a litany of hair-care horrors: Of hot combs dropped on necks. Of sisters almost going out like Van Gogh. Of scalps lined with keloids from countless no-lye, no-lie perms. And of a friend whose father decided to relax her hair himself, leaving her, at age nine, naked and shrieking, almost blinded by the lye, while he went out for a beer."

In one segment of the Rio Hair text, Mary solicits audience members to share *their* painful hair experiences. One woman describes enduring a series of painful injuries. Mary asks her, "You went back for more?" and she answers, "I wanted that look." Mary doesn't ask why. She seems to understand. She proposes that consumers can be spared such pain and indignity by using Rio.

On the website, black women address the role of internalized oppression and the lengths it drives women to as they debate the virtues of Rio and later discuss litigation over its harmful effects. The discussion found in the archives of this online message board provides a glimpse of the complex and often contradictory positions of black women on hair care.

Nancy writes, "O.K.! O.K.! I finally saw the RIO infomercial. I was half asleep and the TV was watching me, when I heard the crowd roar 'RIO.' I saw it at the point when they are stating that 'NOW YOU CAN THROW YOUR HAIR.' Now y'know we are still trying to compete with Miss Barbie. Rio is another way of saying now you too can have White Girl hair and swing it. Pitiful! Peace, Nancy."

A very interesting thread ensues months later when Debbie leaves a message asking for others' opinions regarding Rio and a man, Tbone, responds to her: "I think that Rio is for women of African descent who have an inferiority complex. I think it's for women who want a hair texture that is denatured (no proteins) and mutated. You know, like White women's hair." Though TBone points out the internalized oppression operating here, he does so in a sexist, judgmental way, ironically exercising the prerogative of men to judge women on the level of physical appearance, which only serves to deepen the "inferiority complex" to which he refers.

Victoria responds to Tbone: "I think that RIO or any product is for any woman who wants to do whatever she wishes with 'her' hair. If the sister wishes to braid it up, so be it, if she wishes to straighten it, so be it, if she wishes to shave it all off and go bald, that is her prerogative, as it is her hair. Hair is a woman's crown, how she chooses to arrange that crown does not indicate any sense of inferiority. Is a White woman who curls, straightens, pads, or weaves her hair feeling inferior?"

I wouldn't say "inferior," but we white women do feel insecure about our looks, especially as we compete with other white women. We never feel like we measure up, either—though we have no idea what it feels like to live with the kind of racist and sexist pressure surrounding black women's hair.

VIRGIN HAIR

Mothers face a highly charged decision as they weigh whether to relax their daughter's hair or not. Hair-product manufacturers certainly make it tempting enough by touting the mildness of their kiddie perms. Dark-N-Lovely's Beautiful Beginnings promises "A Wonderful Start for Beautiful Hair . . . The Safest, Gentlest Children's Relaxer." Andre assures his audience that Rio works as well on the daughter's hair as it does on the mother's: "In Brazil," he says, "the mothers put it on their children and have them go out and play in the sun all day long."

> *I remember the first time I was struck by the difference in the hair of black people and white people. I was very young, and a black woman named Alberta took care of me. I loved the smell and energy of her home, with its dark wood and big, heavy furniture. Of her daughters, Toni and Dale were my favorites. Often they would surround me and ask to "play with my hair." At first this seemed unremarkable, but then I began to realize that the girls had an excessive relish for touching and styling my hair. I knew mine was different from theirs, but I sensed that they liked mine better and wished theirs was more like it. It felt strange to be the object of so much envy and admiration, but I loved the attention.*

On the Afroam online bulletin, little black girls' hair is a big topic. Joyce explains that she knows that she acts on internalized oppression in her treatment of her own hair, but not in her treatment of her daughter's. She writes, "Just an aside on the hair thing . . . I thought for a second about getting RIO for my seven-year-old who wants to let her hair hang free, but I really don't want to put anything in my baby's head that would possibly seep into her brain. I read an article in the Detroit News that when they did autopsies on women who had perms they found the chemicals had gotten into their brain tissue. I have a perm now, not something I regularly do, but . . . I can make all kinds of unhealthy choices for myself, but when it comes to my babies now that's different."

However, later in this same post, Joyce reveals the way she still struggles with how people regard kinky hair: "By the way I am sure many people think my two girls' (ages 7 and 2) hair is unkempt by the end of the week. Their hair is so thick (2-year-old) or long and tangly (7-year-old) that they hate having their hair combed. I don't know how to cornrow, and they are tormented so I try to fix it in a way that I only have to do it once or twice a week. This may sound like child abuse but as long as it doesn't get too bad they are happy."

Interestingly, Nancy, who has been opposed to the oppressive (racist) logic of the Rio commercial, admits that she had been considering Rio for her daughter: "Hey Joyce," she writes, "ship them babies to Iowa and I will cornrow their hair. I had thought about RIO for my 5 yr old for the same reason as yours. We have to hold Kinnethia down and entertain, feed, hold her hand, and give breaks to cornrow [her hair]. The cornrows used to last about 3 weeks but now that her hair has gotten thicker, it fuzzies up in a week. But I can't put chemicals in her hair and I don't want to start pressing her hair just to cornrow it PLUS she still will pitch a fit with that. If anyone else has a shampoo, a hair grease or something to make us mothers happier please put it out or call 1-800-IT-NAPPY— peace, Nancy."

THE COST OF "FREEDOM"

Tens of thousands of black women and girls who used Rio suffered hair loss, watched their hair turn green, and/or endured scalp burns, blisters, and sores. For many, these were the very conditions from which they sought refuge.

A Brazilian company, Declasse Cosmeticos, manufactured the product, which was marketed by a group of companies and individuals in the United States, primarily through the infomercials. While the slick ads claimed the product was natural, Rio Hair Naturalizer contained an unnaturally high acidic level, along with harsh chemicals. One ingredient, cupric chloride acid, was more acidic than is wise even in a heavy industrial product, according to a *Cosmetic Insiders' Report*.

In 1997 California attorney general Daniel E. Lungren ruled against the World Rio Corporation in a class-action suit. "While having green hair or no hair may be the fashion trend for some Californians," Lungren said, "it is a choice to be made voluntarily, not accidentally by the use of a faulty product." The plaintiffs won the lawsuit, and a settlement of $4.5 million was awarded to all who experienced problems with the product and had filed with the court to that effect. Still, after the legal fees were paid, there wasn't much money to go around. And the company, which claimed it was in the red, slunk away. So everybody who filed got a few coins to ease their weary heads.

While the court decision was somewhat consoling to these women, there were more delicate issues that never surfaced during the trial, or in the media coverage of the event. Questions remain like Why is it still necessary for black women to go to such lengths to make their hair "desirable"? How is black women's pain made deeper by betrayals such as the one Rio wrought? And how can the whole notion of what is deemed beautiful be overturned, along with the economic system that drives women to pursue it?

As long as there are profits to be made, however, we will continue to see companies sell promises they can't keep, all the while smacking of racism. Fighting it means that we need to look at the way oppression affects everyone, whether it's based on color, gender, sexual orientation, or class. We must also be aware of how vulnerable we are to the Cinderella claims of infomercials like Rio, and the devastating consequences that are possible when we buy a flawed dream marketed to us in a pretty package.

A SHORT HISTORY OF EARLY HAIR STRAIGHTENING
Willie Morrow

Before the black beauty-culture pioneers developed the hot comb, black women used to groom, straighten, and curl their hair in resourceful, and often ingenious, ways, using readily available materials.

The hair was cleaned by techniques such as weaving cotton through the prongs of a table fork and combing the hair with the fork to remove dust and dirt. Chopped corn was rubbed into the hair for the same purpose. Kerosene was used to dry-clean the hair by rinsing it through the hair repeatedly, or applying the kerosene to a rag and rubbing the rag over strands of hair. Or kerosene and turpentine would be mixed with butter or lard and combed through the hair. Wood coals from the fire were rubbed against small strands of hair as a cleanser and deodorizer.

Rainwater was collected for shampoos, and dishwater was used to rinse the hair, since it was believed that the nutrients in the dishwater would be good for the hair. Laundry bluing was used as a rinse to soften the hair and accent its texture. Some enslaved women used freshly churned butter or mutton tallow as a hair conditioner. This created problems, however, since animal fats attracted flies and became rancid and foul-smelling after a while. A unique hair and skin conditioner was wild apple leaves and chicken fat boiled together.

The house workers also introduced the European comb to the field workers. The teeth, however, broke off in thick, woolly hair that might have gone months or years without being combed. Both house and field workers looked for methods to make the hair smoother and more manageable. Black women who worked in the master's house often combed the hair of the master's children while their own children looked on. Some pointed out to their children that the white children never cried when their hair was being groomed, possibly the roots of the concept "tenderheaded."

Hair-straightening techniques included wrapping the hair around a hot knife and pressing the hair with the small irons used for smoothing clothes.

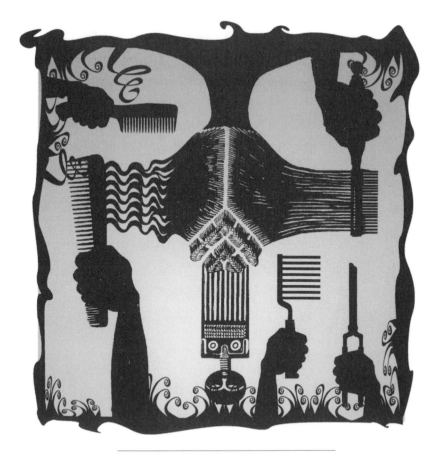

Pen-and-ink line drawing.

DANIEL MINTER

The irons were heated on a stove or in the fireplace and pressed against the hair, which was spread out on the flat surface where the head rested. Sometimes pieces of coarse cloth were heated on top of the stove and pressed against the hair.

Some methods and implements of hair care were quite crude. One was to smear the heavy axle grease from wagons over the hair. The grease was so stiff that it could only be put on the hair, not worked into it. Brushing the stiff hair straightened it out into a flat style. Axle grease, however, proved to be more of a hindrance than a help. The brushing that followed the application of heavy grease stretched the hair beyond its endurance, and the hair broke off in bunches. The only way axle grease could be removed from the hair was with a strong lye solution, which caused additional damage to the hair and created some scalp problems.

Applying hog lard to the hair created a similar problem. The lard would pick up so much dirt and grit that it became difficult, if not impossible, to remove, even with strong grease cutters such as lye soap. In fact, the lye soap often became a part of the thick, greasy film instead of removing it.

Some enslaved black people were able to use blacksmith materials in creating the prototype of the straightening comb, and early formulas concocted in the yard serve as the basic elements of modern hair relaxers.

To make lye soap hair straightener, ashes from the fireplace were collected and put in a pot with a small hole at the bottom. Water was poured in, and a chemical known as potash would then drip down, one drop at a time. The potash could dissove animal bone and fat, and became known after the Civil Was as potash lye. This method was first used to help make soap.

Once mixed, the lye was poured over hog lard and tallow, plus other unusable animal

▪ late 1950s ▪

The hair of colored girls in steaming NYC, Jersey, and Philly ghettos in the summers of the late 1950s were harbingers of the popular "bouffant" hairstyles of the early 1960s. Soon the sisters were emulating Jackie Kennedy's teased and sprayed emulations of what their straightened hair looks like when it starts to go back. Then the Ronnettes of Spanish Harlem exaggerated the bouffant beehive look big-time, and Motown's wiggery capped it.

parts, stirred, and left to set. The lye would dissolve the bones, and a cakelike block would form. The lye soap was mixed with water, butter, potatoes, and lard to make the first "relaxer."

SAY AMEN, SOMEBODY

The names of these beauty shops in the Washington, D.C., area say it all: Deliverance Beauty Salon, Divine Design, and Christ Did it All Beauty Salon, among others. In one, seven women in a circle clasp hands, bow their heads and pray. "Tears trickled down one woman's face as she bellowed a cascade of praises in tongues. With that, the group fell silent. Now it was time to do hair."
—A report on the rise in Christian-themed beauty shops,
Washington Post, 1999

SET IT OFF

Black chorus girls in the 1921 hit Broadway musical *Shuffle Along* were the original flappers and helped to ignite the bobbed-hair trend. As a reporter in the entertainment trade paper *Variety* observed, "Broadway may not know it but the fashion of wearing the feminine head with the bobbed hair effect has more fully invaded the high browns of the colored troupes than in the big musical shows."

ALL-TIME TOP HAIR DIVAS

Jenyne Raines

These style-setters have swung, locked, and chopped their manes for change.

Josephine Baker. La Baker popularized the sleek, short cut with the kewpie-doll curl over each ear. Her glossy, close cropped 'do epitomized the insouciance of the Roaring Twenties—jazzy and care-free.

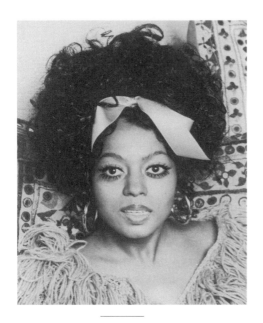

Diana Ross.

PHOTOFEST

Etta James. With don't-bit-mo'-care-what-chu-think flair, the rockin' rhythm-and-blues queen was one of the first black women entertainers to bleach and blond her hair. She flung open a door to the light that Dinah Washington and other black women of every hue would stream through.

Diana Ross. The supreme icon worked the flip and the inflated bouffant into our collective consciousness. The Boss's favorite 'do, the long curly mane, comes with its own fan for that glamorous wind-blown look.

Pat Evans. A '70s model, Pat made bald sexy two decades before Michael Jordan got with it. Elegant, jaw-dropping, stunning, Pat's nude noggin was accentuated by lush lashes and large earrings.

Cicely Tyson. This actress boldly appeared on TV with a short natural at a time when black people on the tube were so rare that a sighting was occasion to summon

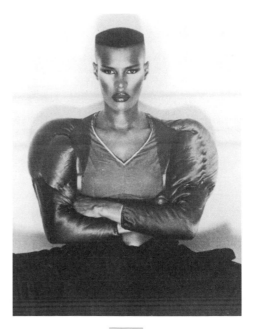

Grace Jones.

PHOTOFEST

everybody in the house. Later appearing at galas in elegantly styled cornrows, Tyson was the first celebrity to demonstrate that the country style could go Hollywood.

Grace Jones. The model-turned-chanteuse-turned-living-work-of-art introduces the severely sculpted natural, known as the fade.

Oprah Winfrey. The Queen of Talk is the talk of the sisters with her thick, bouncy, shoulder-length layered cut. Sans wig or weave, Oprah set the standard for beautiful, healthy hair—that moves!

Whoopi Goldberg. Actress, comedian and iconoclast, the Whoopster brings her locks onto the silver screen and becomes one of the highest paid black actresses of all time. Whoopi's success is all the more exciting because her nap-happy hair challenged the notion of what a black movie star should look like.

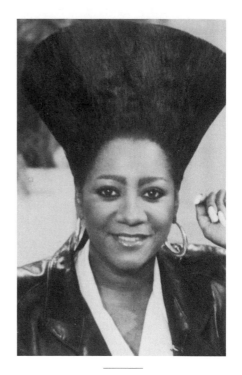

Patti Labelle.

PHOTOFEST

Patti Labelle. Like her staggering voice, the R&B songbird's sculpted hair styles have the power to scream and astound.

Anita Baker, Halle Berry and Toni Braxton. This trio diverted our attention from long hair with their pixie cuts. No longer a crime in the community, short hair was bigtime sharp, carefree chic, and all-time sassy.

Naomi Campbell. The princess of black models clinched her title with Rapunzel hair. Stalking the catwalks with unabashedly long, sleek hair, the leggy British supermodel brought the weave stage front and center.

Mary J. Blige. The hip-hop soul singer reignited blond ambition by sporting various golden tones, lengths and styles, sometimes all in the same week!

Lil' Kim. The pint-sized rapper rocks a wig with sassy aplomb, be it brassy Mae West blond or a lavender china chop.

TONSORIAL PLEASURES

A celebration of the brothers who compete with the divas strand for strand.

Cab Calloway. Mr. Hi-De-Hi-De-Ho's seal-slick conk was the epitome of craazeey cool.

Clarence Williams III. Better known as "Linc" in the late sixties TV series *The Mod Squad,* brotherman was the first to charge the small screen with a superbad bush and smoldering intensity.

The Jackson Five and the Sylvers. Bubblegum loverboys thrilled us with their syncronized moves, tightass bellbottoms, and towering 'fros.

Ron O'Neal. Super Fly was indeed that. Priest's soft, shoulder-skimming hair was the envy of the ghetto dandies.

Big Daddy Kane. Ain't no half-steppin with the rapper's signature high-top fade. Kane's chiseled hair and ebony face made him the prince of darkness.

Snoop Dog. A hair chameleon, the Long Beach-based rapper could have been a tonsorial model. A big 'fro today, thick cornrows tomorrow, two braids Thursday, and Shirley Temple curls on Friday, yet he still manages to come off as a man's man.

Prince. A direct descendant of Cab and Ron O'Neal, the entertainer has gone through some 'dos, but seems to favor straight, touchable hair. Whether he's in a well-coiffed curl or is giving up a sexy shag with the ends tipped in black, this doe-eyed dish appeals to all tastes.

Dennis Rodman. The blushing bride is as color-crazy as he wants to be. Platinum, green or purple, the Rod Man believes in standing out, as if being 6'5" isn't enough.

Maxwell. For-tu-nate to behold that postmodern 'fro on top of the maximum lover. The unruly shock of hair shows just how wild Maxwow is for the ladies.

Latrell Sprewell and Alan Iverson. Old-school fine with ruff neck flava, Spree and Ive fuse the tender and the tough with their designer cornrows.

Wrappers' Delight

We've been wrapping for centuries. In Africa, string-wrapped hair creates all-over-the-head spokes and loops and sculptural sensations. Over here, during slavery, strips of rags, wrapped round the hair, straightened the kinks, while scarves and turbans kept the sweat off the brow and made Mammy presentable to the folks in the big house. More recently, wrapping prepped you for a Black Panther party or symbolized a type of music called Baduizm. Covering the head has always been a sign of deference to God, whether worn by sisters in the church or in the mosque.

HOW TO WRAP A GELE

Start with a large square piece of sturdy fabric such as 100 percent cotton. (Tie-dyed cotton works well!) Fold the cloth diagonally to make a triangle. (If your hair is long, pull it back into an elastic ponytail holder.) Drape the fabric along the front hairline, pull the two ends back under the tuft of hair in back, and bring them around to the front, wrapping one over the other, and then tucking the ends inside. Now you're good to go.

—Akissi Britton

When folks need the basics of life
Do they care
About what's under the head wraps or turbans
That I wear?

—Mildred E. Nero-Drinkard

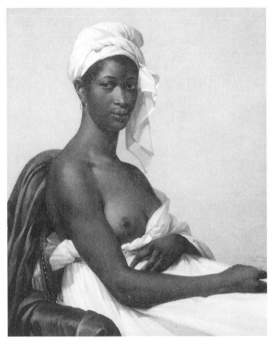

SOFT SCULPTURE

*Portrait of a "Négresse" ca. 1800 from the
Louvre, Paris, France.*

ERICH LESSING/ART RESOURCE

Erykah Badu, 1990s, United States.

DANNY CLINCH/OUTLINE

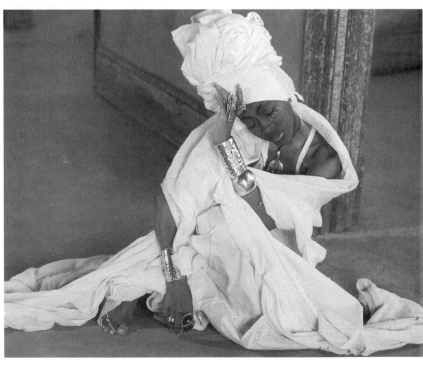

UNDER COVER
Halima Taha

There are said to be more than 100,000 veils between God and His Creation. As I considered writing about my hair, I asked myself, How do I describe my experience without unveiling the subject? As a Muslim woman, how do I speak publicly about that which is supposed to remain private? These concerns are ever-present as I evolve in my understanding about what it means to veil my hair within the spiritual and physical world in which I live.

In the days before I became a believer, I, like many American women, thought Islam was an antiquated religion that oppressed and degraded its female followers, though nothing I had read in the Qur'an substantiated this perception. I assumed that when Muslim women concealed their outer beauty, they forfeited

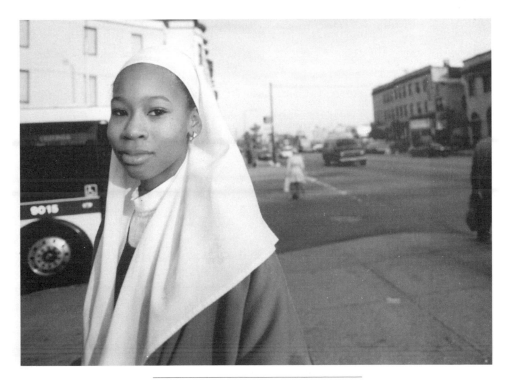

Woman in Muslim wrap on New York street.

LINDA DAY CLARK

sexuality, individuality, and progressive thought. Images of Afghan, Saudi, and Iranian women clad in black from head to toe with face veils only reinforced my perceptions.

As I moved further toward Islam, this confusion began to clear. I soon realized that the oppressive and inhumane treatment of Muslim women is more reflective of compulsive cultural traditions and the media than actual Islamic law. In 1993 I became a practicing Muslim (one who submits to the will of Allah—Arabic for God), and embraced Islam (peaceful submission) as a way of life.[1] In a society that accentuates hair and fashion as adornment, a social passport, and sexual appeal, I choose to conceal my hair. This decision has enabled me to make profound discoveries about self-love, liberation, and the politics of hair.

In retrospect, I realized that before I began to cover my tresses, I received a steady stream of confusing messages about the importance of hair.

I remember being eight years old, in my grandmother's kitchen in Harlem, marveling as she made Mrs. Jenkins's hair sail through the teeth of a hot comb without touching the surface beneath her hairline. Eagerly, I looked forward to Grandma's final parting curl by swinging my patent leather feet, like a pendulum beneath my chair, in anticipation of skipping away from the aroma of pressed hair.

One Sunday my shiny shoes caught Mrs. Jenkins's eye as she and my grandmother swapped opinions on celebrities, politics, and men. Mrs. Jenkins motioned me toward her with the promise of the peppermints in her hand.

"Lord have mercy, girl, you sure are pretty," she exclaimed. "Look at that beautiful head of hair. You don't know how fortunate you are to be blessed with such good hair."

This was the first time I had ever heard of good hair. Isn't all girls' hair good, I thought, when clean, combed, and braided? But from Mrs. Jenkins's excitement, it became apparent that some girls, just by virtue of the hair they were born with, would never have merited her enthusiasm.

When I was twelve, my mother and I attended a weekend conference spon-

---

[1] My understanding that there is no deity but God is affirmed by rising before dawn to observe the first of five daily prayers; fasting for the month of Ramadan; undertaking the Hajj pilgrimage to Mecca at least once in a lifetime; and paying the zakat or charity, which requires faith, sincerity and self-discipline in my daily actions.

sored by the National Black Feminist Organization. The culmination of the event for me, as the youngest participant, was being invited to contribute an essay to *Ms.* magazine. Giddy with delight, I felt ushered into the ranks of womanhood. But my mother, who embraced James Brown's "I'm Black and I'm Proud" as her personal anthem, intimated that I hadn't gone far enough. She suggested that I cut my hair into an Afro as a symbolic rite of passage.

I was dumbfounded. My hair was already in its natural state. How would cutting it make me any more black, female, or political? Besides, I cherished the Sunday-night hair-combing rituals my mother and I shared. They were filled with talk and TV and the sharp scents of Hair So New and No More Tears. My favorite moment was when my mother carefully put the rubber bands on the ends of my braids, took one in each hand, and gently pulled me toward her for my good-night kiss. Still, my mother persisted, with the best of intentions. So, reluctantly, I followed her lead and let my tresses be snipped and fluffed until a curly Afro stood in the place of my braids.

My Puerto Rican, Irish, African, and Jewish girlfriends continued to appreciate my friendship. But when the black girls in my class saw my new 'fro they were disgusted and angry. I naively had no idea that something so basic to the human body would provoke such strong emotions. They completely stopped talking to me and began to whisper and snicker behind my back as we walked the hallways between classes. In the girls' bathroom they scribbled insults under my name like:

Stupid bitch, don't you want to be beautiful!

and

Fluff Puff thinks she's tuff.

The ultimate humiliation, though, was being shunned from sitting with them at "our" table—simply because I had cut my hair. In the sad six months that followed the powerful National Black Feminist Conference, I thought I had hit bottom. My "sistas" gave me cause to worry about the future of black women. But my hair woes only worsened as I became a woman, and men began to impose their hair obsessions on me as well.

Still, in the early days of concealing my hair, even as I escaped the pressures of others' expectations, I felt wedged between two worlds. For many years I was a dancer and model who thrived on being applauded for how I moved. The dancer in me still saw the body as an instrument for movement and form. As I progressed deeper into Islam, I had to explore how to move without objectifying my body. Since I had begun modeling at fourteen, I had become accustomed to being appreciated for the contours of my face and frame. I had been a part of a world that believes the ability to turn heads is proportional to self-worth. While I intuitively recognized the distorted relationship between beauty and feminine value in our culture, I still wanted it both ways—to be admired for my looks and to be respected for who I really was.

The Prophet Muhammad, the "last messenger of God"—may peace and blessings be upon Him—was among the earliest reformers on behalf of women. At a time when women in all parts of the world were repressed, he said that it is a God-given right for a woman to inherit and bequeath property, to seek knowledge, to choose marriage and/or divorce, and to exercise full possession and control over her own wealth. He upheld the Qur'an's abolishment of such sex-discriminating practices as female infanticide, slavery, and levirate (marriage between a man and his brother's widow).

Still, early in my journey, I couldn't foresee how covering the female body served to cherish it for a higher spiritual purpose rather than mere self-display. I struggled to understand how safeguarding the soul enhances one's humanity. Gradually, I discovered that the beautiful energy of my feminine physique, when covered, has the potential to radiate a more profound message about my deeper identity rather than extinguish it. Today I fully appreciate the Islamic concept of womanhood—"a female human being with her own soul"—versus the Judeo-Christian notion of a woman being "of/for man."

My journey of self-discovery involved, in part, learning how to cover yet still have my own style. This process was new and unfamiliar. In pursuit of pleasing my Creator, while maintaining my individuality, I explored hats, hats with scarves, and scarves by themselves. Using streams of colorful fabric, I made twisted sculpture and knotted mountains. It took me a while, but soon I began to realize that the reflection in my mirror revealed not only a pallete of fluid hues and shapes but the cheery face of that contented eight-year-old in my grandmother's kitchen.

From the first day I wrapped my head, I experienced a renewed personal freedom. I began to joyfully experience myself from the inside out. Shielding me from the harshness of the world, covering my hair cultivated personal intimacy, taking me further into a new world of privacy, security, and peace. It increased my self-awareness and became a buffer between me and the misogynist society in which all women live.

Shortly after I began to cover my hair, I meandered through the Metropolitan Museum of Art. I looked for Christian and Jewish pictorial representations of earlier prophets and the women of those times. From the dawn of civilization, head scarves and flowing dresses have always been associated with "Godliness" or "God consciousness." This origin can be traced to early Christianity and Judaism, when these religions were in their purest form of practice.[2]

This tradition is reflected in the Qur'an, wherein Allah says, "O Children of Adam! We have bestowed raiment upon you to cover yourselves and as an adornment. But the raiment of righteousness that is better" (7:26) and "O Prophet, tell your wives and daughters and the believing women, that they should cast their outer garments over their persons (when out of doors): that is most convenient, that they should be known (as such) and not molested. And Allah is Oft-Forgiving, Most Merciful" (33:59).

Being a Muslim woman is not all about clothes and covering up. There is an inner as well as an outer covering. Combined, these two provide peace of mind and heart. My spiritual consciousness manifests through my actions, which include my behavior, speech, and appearance in public. My demeanor symbolizes the exalted status we were created to have as women. Though primarily an inner journey, the changes in my outer appearance have drawn a reaction from friends and colleagues: *Halima, what on earth did you do with your hair? . . . Girrrl, I know you didn't cut your hair! Did you? . . . What possessed you to cover your hair like that? . . . Well, you look good, though. You really do!*

---

[2] In the Bible it states, "But any woman who prays and prophecies with her head unveiled dishonors her—it is the same as if her head were shaven, for if a woman will not veil herself, then she should cut off her hair. But if it is disgraceful for a woman to be shorn or shaven, let her wear a veil" (1 Corinthians 11:5). Orthodox Jewish women veil based on the MinHartorah for married women (or a woman who was married in the past—MB75:11) to have her hair covered whenever she is in public areas or appears among a large number of people. This is derived from the verse "The Kohen shall uncover the hair of the Sotah" (Brnidbar 5:1)

Casual acquaintances pried deeper: *What's under there? . . . Can I see? . . . Can I touch?* As well as: *There's something different about you. I'm not quite sure what it is, though. You look very comfortable and peaceful.*

Many times people asked and answered their own questions as I listened. Ironically, they would see something positive in me, but still needed to mentally contradict the visible affirmation of what they felt. It was as if covering my hair or dressing more modestly couldn't possibly look or feel as good as it does. In the same breath, however, they would say, "You look beautiful!"

Some of the most unexpected responses came from women I had never met before. They have chased me down the street, held open closing New York City subway doors, cornered me in public rest rooms, and craned their necks over crowds on opposing escalator stairs, simply to ask, "Where did you purchase your fabric?" "Why do you cover your head?" "Could you show me how to do that?" Or pointing with fascination to my head: "Is that a spiritual thang?" The best part of this public affirmation is that I have met some wonderful and interesting women simply because they were interested in how and why I covered my hair.

Although my covering does not prohibit men from being attracted to me as a woman, it definitely alters the way they approach me. My allure now seems more human, removing sex from the appeal. Interacting with me in the workplace, men are more respectful, professional, and better focused on business. Men who don't know me tend to be more courteous. And much to my delight, the harassing cat-calls and personal remarks have largely been silenced. Perhaps this is because people instinctively show deference to a covered woman—witness the respect paid to nuns.

In an era when sexual harassment has become lawfully prohibited as a public policy, I have found an effective personal way to uphold and defend my honor and integrity and shield myself from exploitation. It facilitates free movement in society and serves as a practical symbol of liberation.

Covered, I feel as if I am raised from the inelegant to the gracious, from the showpiece to the refined, and from the everyday to the special. The spiritual intention behind veiling my hair has purged me of the notion that I have to be publicly displayed to be noticed and known. I can now aspire to the best within myself.

As a wife, I never imagined that being covered in public and unveiling myself in the private security of my home could so dramatically keep my marriage as exciting and delightful as it has. Whenever I see my husband, I enjoy a new feeling of excitement, as if we are meeting for the first time. In covering myself from public scrutiny, I am able to more meaningfully share myself with him. The intimacy between us is precious and exclusively ours. All veils between us are cast aside.

For me, Islam was my first step toward liberation from practices that stifle spirit within every community. To me, the effect of the Western model of womanhood is akin to a straitjacket. It imposes dysfunctional prototypes for blackness, beauty, femininity and acceptability. I no longer cry for my "sista friends." Instead I pray for them, knowing that their highest good is well within reach. By directing our concerns away from the politics of fashion and hair to being caretakers of our own integrity, dignity, and self-respect, we can cherish what is most precious—ourselves.

One evening, while contemplating this essay, I dined with my husband, a family friend, and his associate. Over the course of the meal, I reflected on men, in general, and my husband in particular. Glancing around the room, it seemed to me that the men in the restaurant represented a microcosm of all the men I have ever known. And in their diversity and splendor, it became clear to me that behind the nice clothes, cologne, smile, and talk, there is always the man who desires the woman all of the time, covered and uncovered. And then there is the man who is seeking the woman, not to unveil her but to know her. I felt a smile spread across my face like a slow sunrise, warming me with happiness. I realized that I am blessed to be married to a man who can truly appreciate the depths of my mind, body, and spirit.

As I savored the moment, the maître d' escorted a well-groomed eight-year-old-boy to the table. Shyly approaching me as the ambassador for his family from across the room, he asked, "Miss, are you a princess?" My friends were amused. My husband glanced at me and quietly rejoiced in the secrets we share. I smiled at him, and then answered graciously, "No, I am not a princess, I am a woman."

TALKING HEADS

In Martinique and Guadeloupe in the eighteenth and nineteenth centuries, the ways in which women's heads were wrapped and tied symbolized status, occupation, personality, and disposition. "Styles of headgear were fixed by tradition

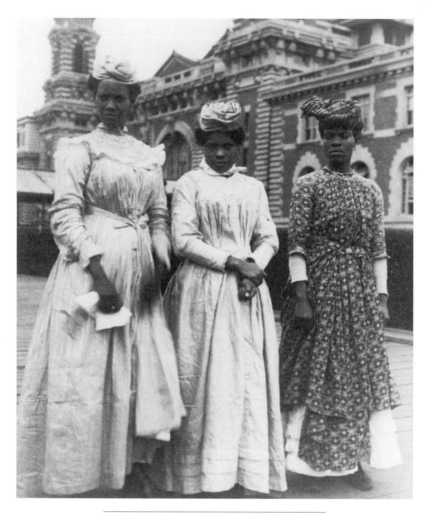

Women from Guadeloupe arriving at Ellis Island.

SCHOMBURG CENTER FOR RESEARCH IN BLACK CULTURE

for the cane-cutter, the laundress, the courtesan, the nurse, the field worker, and the house servant. Personal style and whim decreed the subtle variations in each design." The tilt of a headwrap, as well as the number of points in it, communicated "mood, marital status or availability."

—Grazielle Bontemps with Anca Bertrand, *Coifs et Coiffures de la Martinique*

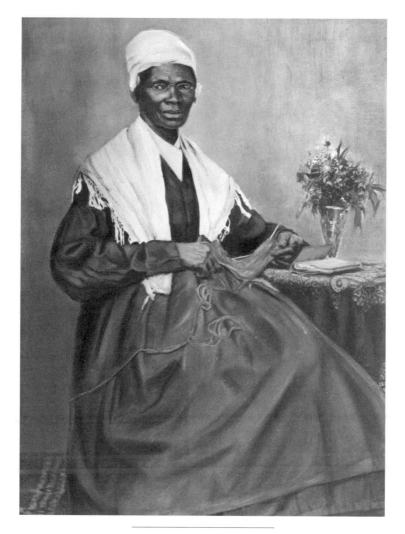

Sojourner Truth: head bound, mind free.

BETTMAN/CORBIS

STRINGING US ALONG

Among black women in the rural South, the practice of "wrapping" the hair with thread or string continued into the early twentieth century. When store-bought thread was not available, women used the white string from cotton bags, tobacco vines, or strips of stockings to wrap hair that had been oiled with lard or fatback grease. Keeping springy hair elongated and untangled, the technique somewhat smoothed the kinks.

Memories of enslaved women's string-wrapped hair evoked joy in Peter Clifton: "I meets Christina and seek her out for to marry. Dere was somethin' about dat gal dat day I meets her, though her hair had about a pound of cotton thread in it, dat just attracted me to her like a fly will sail 'round and light on a 'lasses pitcher."

GRANDMA BLOWS HER TOP
Gloria Wade Gayles

My grandmother had seen so much racial violence in her younger days that she became one of those "bad colored women," the kind so angry that they are crazy enough to be crazy around white folks. That was my grandmother—a formidable opponent when she chose to be. I was with her the day a white clerk called her "nigger" in the downtown Woolworth's, an identity visible only because I was with her. She reached for a hammer

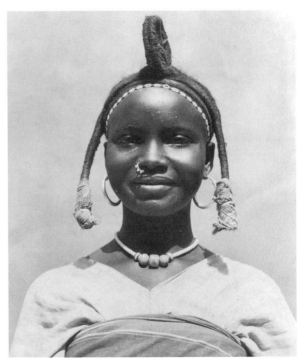

Sudanese beauty with string-wrapped hair.

BETTMAN/CORBIS

that was lying on the counter and brandished it. "I'll bash your head in, woman," she said. "Do you hear me. I'll bash your head in." God, but she was beautifully tough.

On the day that stands out most vividly in memory, she was with me downtown at Goldsmith's shopping in preparation for Easter. I was perhaps seven. Then black people could not drink from water fountains except those in the basement (where the water was never cool) or use rest rooms except those in the basement (where there were no doors to the stalls). And we could not try on hats. The grease from our hair would soil the merchandise, "they" claimed.

On this day, Grandmama and I were on the third floor. She was busy studying dresses. I use "studying" for a reason: she would look closely at how the dresses were put together, fingering every seam and looking, with gifted eyes, at every stitch. Then she would return home to re-create that which she had studied. She would place newspaper on the kitchen table and cut pattern pieces from memory, freehand. She would pin the pieces to the fabric, also placed on the kitchen table, and cut them with perfection. I remember her sitting for hours working the treadle on the old machine that sat to the right of the kitchen door. She would not move until she had finished, all except for the hem, an enviable copy of the original.

Whenever I shopped with her, I would have time to be mischievous because she was busy "studying." That is what happened on the day of the incident. She was busy, and I was mischievous. I put on a pretty pink bonnet. Immediately, the white saleslady jerked it off my head and said loudly to my grandmother, "You know better'n let this nigger put on a hat in *this* store." Within seconds, my grandmother went into action. She ordered me to put the bonnet on again. With tightened lips, she told the saleslady, "Now touch it. Just touch it."

Perhaps it was my grandmother's near-white complexion (she often passed when doing so benefited her family) or the intensity of her rage that froze the saleslady in an expression of, first, surprise, and then fear. My grandmother said again, with tighter lips, "Just touch it." The saleslady did not move. I modeled the hat as my grandmother instructed. "Turn around, Gloria Jean," she told me. "Let's see." I twirled a bit.

- 1920s -

A NIGHT CAP

An ad in the *Chicago Defender* newspaper says the Europeans invented what big mama's discarded stocking, knotted at one end, was already being used for: "The Ideal hair dressing cap for ladies and gentlemen. A recent European invention, makes the most rebellious hair keep its good appearance. Preserves the coiffure after arranging. Keeps the hair exactly as you want it. No chance to rumple, knot or snarl. Makes unruly hair lie flat. Gives the fashionable straight effect. Excellent for bobbed hair. Indispensable after shampooing. Nothing better for the training and care of children's hair. An absolutely necessary aid to hair beauty."

After we had tasted victory for a few minutes, my grandmother said, "Take it off. It's not pretty enough for you."

UPLIFT
Liddy Jones

Nanette was still running her tongue over her teeth, savoring the chocolate ear of a hollow Easter bunny, as she sat in the fifth pew from the pulpit. Her older sister was singing a solo in the junior choir, and her cousin had written a poem for the risen Jesus. Sitting so close, Nanette should have been able to see everything, but her view was blocked by the hats bobbing and fluttering before her. Flowers, beads, and veils encircled some. Swooping feathers, looping ribbons, and pleated fans festooned others. One brim had a black velvet bird perched on a swirl of pink tulle.

Mrs. Ondine Beasley wore the grandest hat in the whole congregation, and this Sunday her ample body was seated directly in front of Nanette. As the sermon progressed and the reverend's words began to slur, curving around to hoarse harrumphs, Sister Beasley rocked with the rhythms of the Holy Ghost. Her head rolled forward, and then tipped back, forward and then back. Nanette thought the woman was drifting off to sleep. Then she heard the whoop—"Thank ya, Jesus. Thank ya, Lord"—and saw Sister Beasley's hand fly up and freeze in midair. A nurse rushed over to fan the woman. But it was too late. Sister Beasley's hat had been launched.

It sailed high into the air over the sea of hats, and finally Nanette could see.

FOR A JOB WELL DONE

A folk expression for an obsequious black person is "handkerchief head." The term may have been originally coined to refer to the bandanna-wrapped heads of women, and then later to denote the servile behavior of plantation blacks that was rewarded by whites. According to historian Anna Atkins Simkins, on Barbados plantations, bandannas or headkerchiefs were used as rewards for slaves. This custom was also observed on southern plantations.

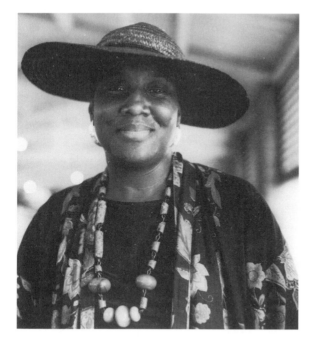

Beaming in a black straw hat.

DEBORAH EGAN,
ALLFORD/TROTMAN

*Hats off to Killer Joe. A 1938
caption to this photo read,
"Whether it is in the boxing ring or
the horse show ring, Joe 'Brown
Bomber' Louis, heavyweight cham-
pion of the world, is always assured
of enthusiastic support."*

UPI/CORBIS-BETTMAN

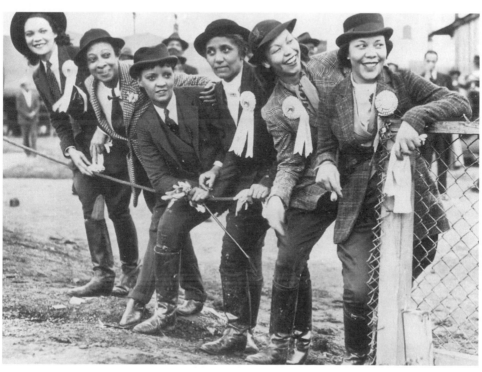

TURBAN RENEWAL

In South Carolina, in the time of slavery, the head mammy in charge wore a crisp white turban to signify her elevated status. While the other house help could wear any colored headrag, Mammy's was only white, and always freshly laundered and sparkling. Her covered head made her acceptable to serve in white folks' most elegant settings. And it eased the discomfort associated with Mammy's blackness.

The women of South Carolina often carried baskets of rice and laundry atop their turbans.

BANDANNA

Michael D. Harris

Aunt Jemima's been the leading handkerchief head for 150 years. At various times she's been a black man in drag, a white man in drag, and an angry black woman with accounts to settle. Through it all, she's remained one of America's most popular advertising symbols, conjured quickly by her bandanna.

Chris L. Rutt, one of the owners of the Pearl Milling Company, developers of a ready-mix pancake flour, got the idea for Aunt Jemima as a living-product trademark in 1889 when he visited a minstrel show in St. Joseph, Missouri. He saw a performance of the cakewalk to the song "Old Aunt Jemima," written by

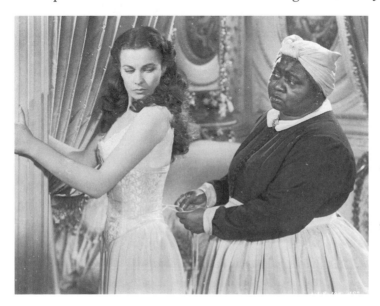

Hattie McDaniel's Academy award-winning mammy from Gone with the Wind.

PHOTOFEST

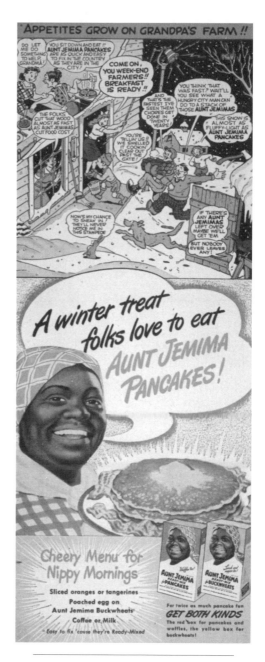

- 1882 -

Author and former abolitionist Frederick Douglass's first wife, Anna, a black woman who wore her hair in a bandanna, was not able to fashion an appearance commensurate with the august reputation of her husband. Historian Arna Bontemps says that in the wake of Anna's death, the expressions that filled Douglass's mail "often struck a quaint note. Old companions of the abolitionist tried to incorporate all their impressions of the naive woman in comments about her good cooking, her tidy house and the appealing picture she made with her head tied in a bandanna. Few of them succeeded in hiding a still stronger feeling that her death revived: admiration for Douglass who, while outgrowing Anna, had never so much as hinted that he felt unequally yoked." A year and a half later, Douglass became the first prominent African American to marry a Caucasian when he wed the woman who had been his secretary in his government post. The new Mrs. Douglass's head, no doubt, was unencumbered.

Advertisement for Aunt Jemima Pancake mix, ca. 1948.

THE GRANGER COLLECTION

Billy Kersands, a black man who was one of the most famous minstrels of his day. Many whites had also performed the popular song, modifying the lyrics. The man Rutt saw that day was a white man in blackface and drag. Wearing an apron and a bandanna, he pretended to be a black cook singing a little ditty:

My old missus promise me
Old Aunt Jemima, oh, oh, oh
When she died she'd set me free
Old Aunt Jemima, oh, oh, oh
She lived so long her head got bald
Old Aunt Jemima, oh, oh, oh
She swore she would not die at all
Old Aunt Jemima, oh, oh, oh

The cakewalk was a dance devised by African Americans to spoof the formal promenades of whites through exaggerated gestures. The fact that "Old Aunt Jemima" was performed to a cakewalk suggests that Kersands had modified the song so that beneath the spoof of blacks lay a coded spoof of whites. Signifyin' on the old "missus," he characterized her as being so mean, so committed to keeping black folks in her service, that she would not die, even after her hair fell out! Hair is a woman's crown, a source of great energy and vanity, and yet this woman kept on despite losing hers.

The Aunt Jemima character was first portrayed by a black woman in 1893 at the World's Columbian Exposition in Chicago—also known as the World's Fair. There Nancy Green, a fifty-nine-year-old former domestic, masqueraded as the pancake mammy. She was wildly popular and helped the new product make its way into thousands of American homes. In 1900 more than 80 percent of the Negro women in Chicago worked as domestics. As they went about their count-less daily chores, many wore headscarfs to cover their hair, which they had no time to style. But the bandanna'd image that Green displayed at the fair was not how they presented themselves in public. Virtually all photographs of black women outside work or domestic situations during this period show them with their heads uncovered and neatly styled. Later, in the 1940s and 1950s, when my mother-in-law came along, she recalls that she and her sisters were not allowed to be seen outside in a headscarf so as not to be linked to demeaning mammy stereotypes.

For whites the bandanna-bound Jemima was a fond, nostalgic image of black servitude. But she came to signify for us the mask of the darky that blacks often wore to make whites comfortable. When I was growing up in Cleveland, Jemima got tossed around like a rag doll. We snapped on each other by asking, "Ain't jo mama on a pancake box?" To suggest that someone's mother could be tied to the pancake mammy was a humorous absurdity because everyone knew that Aunt Jemima was not real. If our mothers, grandmothers, or aunts wore kerchiefs, we never saw them. For them, the bandanna only served to bind them to the hardships of the past, and distanced Aunt Jemima from the elaborate hair traditions of West African women, of whom they were the stylish descendants. It signified all those conditions white folks imposed with their real oppression and their imagined happy servants.

TEARING OFF THE MASK

During the first decades of this century the bandanna began to vanish from the public realm, even in the Deep South, as black women began to straighten their hair. Still, the mammy icon flourished in the popular media. Movies like *Gone with the Wind* and *Imitation of Life* in the 1930s, and later television shows like *Beulah* in the 1950s, repeatedly depicted black women as devoted, strong, asexual females. As late as the 1950s, black women continued to be hired to make public appearances as Aunt Jemima. However in the 1960s whites began to see televised images of real black women like Rosa Parks and Coretta Scott King in the civil rights struggle, and mammy fantasies began to fade. Still, the Quaker Oats Company, who now owned the Aunt Jemima trademark, continued to capitalize on white fondness for the mammy icon by keeping her on the pancake box. They did, however, respond to changing times and black pressure by somewhat modifying the image on the box.

Aunt Jemima was such a powerful, pervasive caricature that by the 1960s a number of black artists attempted to undermine her image. In 1963, Jeff Donaldson painted Aunt Jemima and the Pillsbury Doughboy, another well-known advertising icon, as adversaries locked in struggle. Donaldson transformed the mammy into an angry black woman and the Doughboy into a policeman—a symbol of white authority. The work predicted that one day black folks' masks would come off, and all the residual anger and resistance would be unleashed in the streets. One year later the first Watts riot proved him correct. Two years later the Black Panther Party formed 500 miles to the north of Watts, in Oakland, California. Donaldson's painting was one of the earliest acknowledgments that the images of black women could be tools in liberation struggles. The women behind the masks were not smiling mammies.

Numerous artists who have used Aunt Jemima as a warrior against her own servile image, including Murry DePillars, Jon Lockard, Betye Saar, and Faith Ringgold, reached back for the bandanna in an effort to put plantation mythologies to rest. In these works the unmasked black woman is so menacing that you wouldn't dare ask her to do a cotton-pickin' thing. And you had better not call her "mammy"! These images were the visual equivalent of signifyin'.

The masculine characteristics of Aunt Jemima in some of the artwork further unmasks Aunt Jemima, symbolically tearing off the bandanna and revealing her transvestite roots. Aunt Jemima was born a minstrel, and minstrels were white males masking themselves as blacks. Often they acted out of a literal transvestism by dressing as black women, as well as a cultural transvestism in the minstrel tradition of white (males) masquerading as blacks. The bandanna had for too many years concealed the fact that Mammy was not a black woman, or even a woman at all. She was a white male minstrel's invention. And our signifying about her has always been loaded with innuendo. Our mothers were

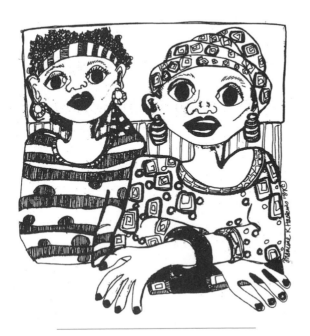

These days, we wrap for style.
Pen-and-ink drawing by Francine Haskins.

not mammies, and Aunt Jemima did not live among us. She lived only in the white imagination. It's all up there under the bandanna.

MAMMY GETS A MAKEOVER

In 1987 the Quaker Oats Company, which now owns the Aunt Jemima trademark, retired her headscarf, gussied her up with a shiny press and curl, and adorned her neck with a lace collar. Still, with her thirty-two-tooth smile, it's not hard to imagine her slipping into a kitchen and whipping up a tall platter of flapjacks. Pass da 'lasses, please.

THE CULTURE OF HAIR SCULPTURE
Juliette Harris

Mirror, mirror on the wall,
Why does my hair snap back into a wiry ball?
What seems like the riddle of nappy hair really is not.
The enigma is easy to figure out if you just think: art!

Kink's acute, complicated curl makes the hair springy and elastic, texturious and thick—qualities perfectly suited for sculpture. Of course kink can be challenging—it will grab on to itself like Velcro and make the most intricate knots known to humanity. But the challenge of animated kink has been the incentive to produce art! Africans carved ornate combs and beautifully patterned, partitioned hairstyles to keep the hair unknotted. While other Africans, like the Masai men, let the knots knit on up in a spiraling dance of life.

African women appreciated the nappy texture and hard density of their hair because these qualities made it capable of being molded into elaborate forms that could speak in all kinds of ways. Theirs were the original "talking heads." African women's hairstyles expressed such things as marital and social status, grief, age, and being an initiate of a particular women's society.

Deeper still, many styles also signaled specific philosophical messages. For example, women in Ghana stressed the importance of knowing about the past by creating a zigzag, cornrowed hairstyle that means "Turn back and get your history." The striking cornrow design depicts the structure of the sankofa bird, whose head points one way while its body points the other.

Eloquent styles were created throughout the continent: patterns of dark, grainy hair against clean, smooth scalp. Artful, articulate geometries. Talk about signifyin'!

Adding to the complexity of African hair sculpture was the environment of love in which the styles were created. While she was living among the Mende women of Sierra Leone, art historian Sylvia Ardyn Boone noticed that to ensure the success of a hairstyle, the working space had to be "cleared of animosities and be full of good will and harmony."

Resettled as slaves in North America, African women did not have the tranquility or luxurious license to leisurely gather and painstakingly beautify one another. Laboring for the master from sunup to sundown and maintaining the slave community from sundown to sleep, women braided their hair in simple plaits or wrapped it with string for maintenance, not style, and covered the entire arrangement with a kerchief or cloth.

Black women living in the lowlands and sea islands of South Carolina, however, were able to retain more African behavior than did black folk living inland. One portrait of a nineteenth-century Sea Island woman depicts a magnificent sculptural hairstyle, including features such as raised, starfish-shaped wedges in the back. This intricate style could only have been created from the type of hair that later generations of black women would bemoan as "coarse."

"Coarse" hair also performed admirably as free black women moved to northern cities and developed fashionable personas. In the 1890s, the popular "Gibson girl" hairstyle worn by white women had a striking counterpart in black women's molded bouffant hairstyles—artfully shaped mounds of smoothed but unstraightened nappy hair. In addition to her crusading journalism, Ida B. Wells was distinguished by her hair, an outstanding example of the molded, kinky style.

While it would be many decades before African-American women would again treat their nappy hair as a sculptural medium, during the intervening years their thick, hot-combed, straightened hair was conducive to molding into the pompadour of the 1940s, the french roll of the late 1950s and early 1960s, the beehive of the early to mid 1960s, and the fantasy, gel-stiffened and rhinestone-studded hairdos of the sistas on the subways in the 1990s. And throughout this period black beauticians excelled in the precision cutting of hair into sharp styles—which indeed is also a form of hair sculpture, as are the creations of braiders who deftly work up wefts of synthetic hair into a wide array of forms.

But nappy hair is most expressive when it speaks in its own voice—without extensions. Today, some of the most impressive cornrow, Nubian knot and twist designs are created through the nimble manipulations of short nappy hair that is just barely long enough to braid or twirl.

And the unrestricted coil of hair itself: pure art. Arrange some naps on a photocopy machine and enlarge them, and enlarge the enlargement, and voilà: a work of art from your hand and the hand of the creator worth framing. The creator wasn't a fool when it came to the design of our hair—the force is the master artist. And so are we when we work with it!

The following examples of nappy-hair artistry over the ages show the infinite versatility of this medium.

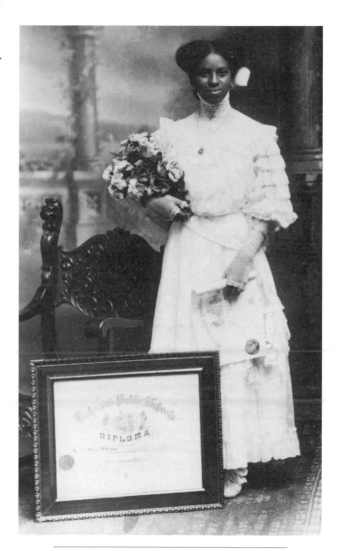

Leonie Helen Holmes is the picture of molded hair perfection in this graduation portrait. Crisp, kinky hair molded into bouffant shapes was worn by African-American women between the 1880s and the 1900s.

COLLECTION VIRGINIA HISTORICAL SOCIETY

▪ 1730s ▪

European explorers to West Africa described a variety of African styles: The hair is "plaited or twisted, and adorn'd with some few trinkets of gold, coral, or glass." They "are very proud of their hair; some wear it in tufts and bunches, and others cut in crosses quite over their heads."

—from *African Textiles and Decorative Arts,*
Roy Sieber

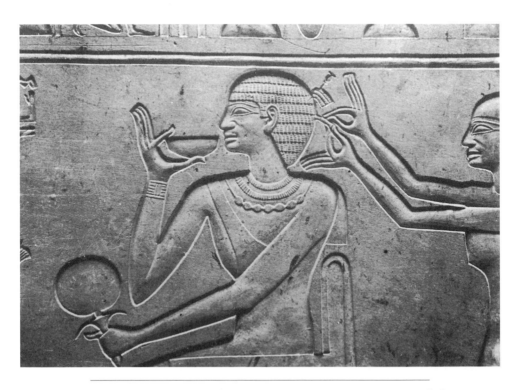

Princess Kiwitt having her hair dressed; a detail from an Egyptian relief.

BETTMAN/CORBIS

EARLY LOCKS

Artists in ancient Greece and Rome admirably depicted the "kinky" texture of African people's hair in portraits of black people on pendants, earrings, necklaces, coins, and pottery. Many images depict a hairstyle consisting of even rows of well-groomed, woolly twists or spirals. Historian Frank Snowden identifies this bronze statuette as perhaps depicting a street singer. It was created circa 200 B.C.

BIBLIOTHÈQUE NATIONALE DE FRANCE

EARLY CORNROWS

Researchers have reported the excavation of the head of a young girl from Nubia (which covered parts of present-day Sudan and Egypt) from around 550–750 A.D. Her hair was braided into cornrows.

—Anna Atkins Simkins, "The Functional and Symbolic Roles of Hair and Headgear Among Afro-American Women: A Cultural Perspective," a Ph. D. thesis.

EARLY BANTU KNOTS

The early European explorers to West Africa were impressed with the coastal people's hair styles. In 1455 the Portuguese explorer Cado Mosto said of the Senegalese, "[Both] sexes . . . weave their hair into beautiful tresses, which they tie into various knots, though it be very short." Two centuries later, another explorer drew the portrait at left of a Gold Coast woman.

BRITISH LIBRARY

EBONY IN IVORY

One of the most elaborate examples of African retention in nineteenth-century African-American hair styling is shown on the ivory bust of Nora August, a former enslaved woman who lived at the Retreat Plantation on St. Simons Island, Georgia. The neckbase of the sculpture is carved with the words: "Nora August, slave, age 23 years. Purchased from the market, St. Augustine, Florida, April 17, 1860. Now a free woman."

The cord-wrapped braid around the front of Nora August's head is exactly like a feature seen in African hair design. The sculpture portrays thick, kinky hair that is divided into five sections and braided into dense, thin rows. Each section is molded into raised, pyramidal-shaped wedges that form a starfish-shaped pattern in back. A U-shaped braid or twist is formed at the nape of the neck.

Presented to the nurses at Darien, Georgia, in 1865, the sculpture, for which Nora August posed, was carved at Retreat Plantation on St. Helena's Island, which was occupied by Union troops and used as an army hospital and camp for contraband slaves. The sculptor may well have been a Union soldier. The portrait of Nora August is a striking representation of African feminine beauty created out of the fusion of a dual inspiration: the artistic imagination of the hair stylist and the inspiration of the sculptor to work a piece of ivory (possibly from Africa and a medium difficult to carve) into fine detail to produce a lasting portrait of a regal, self-possessed, African-featured woman.

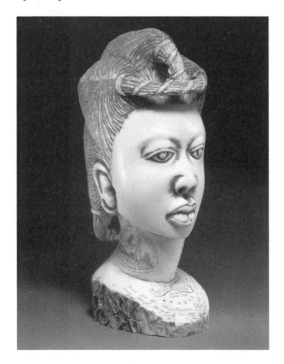

Bust of Nora August.

MUSEUM OF THE CONFEDERACY

SEA ISLAND COMPANY COLLECTION

The rough, bristling texture and animated qualities of kinky hair have long intrigued American artists and illustrators. Contemporary visual artists who have produced works on hair themes include Sonya Clark, David Hammons, Ruth Marten, Alison Saar, Eve Sandler and Lorna Simpson.

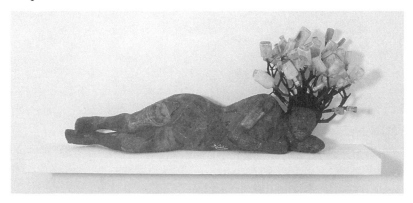

Compton Nocture.
Wood, ceiling tin, bottles.
ALISON SAAR

PHOTO SUPPLIED BY PHYLLIS KIND GALLERY

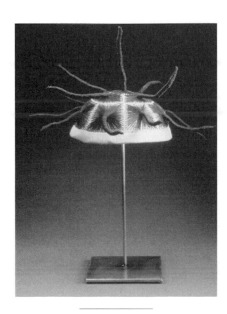

Onigi: 13 Sticks.
Cloth and cotton thread.

SONYA CLARK

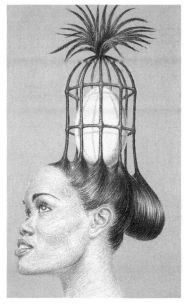

Hairdo.
Gouache and colored pencil.

RUTH MARTEN

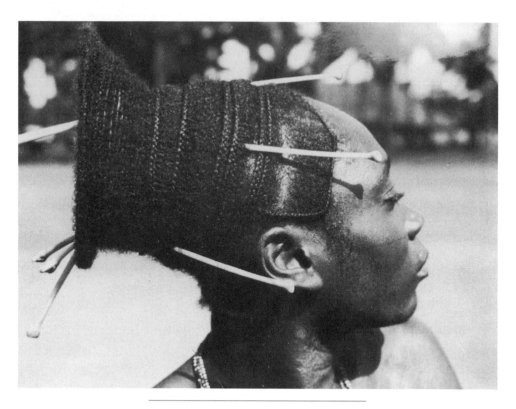

Traditional basket hair style worn by women in the Congo.

▪ 2000 ▪

The Museum for African Art in New York presents the exhibit "Hair in African Art and Culture." In an essay for the exhibit catalog, historian Kennell Jackson discusses the cross-fertilization between contemporary African and African-American hairstyles, as demonstrated on a Harlem shop sign advertising "An African Braid Explosion." The shop offered a full menu of styles, including:

Corkscrews	Box Braids
Flat Twists	Dubie Braids
Corn Rows	Twists Boofruito
Senegalese	Spaghetti Braids
Casamance	African-American Plaits

Pillow Talk

W e try to create hair that is touchable—like the commercials tell us we should—while secretly hoping he won't touch it. Often our hair is an illusion—a look achieved with gobs of gook, or an imported tress, stitched in like the hem of a dress. A guise we put on and take off. Intimacy is a high price to pay for it.

LOVE ADVICE FROM THE EBONY ADVISOR

In the September 1988 issue of *Ebony* magazine, a woman sought counsel from the publication's "Ebony Advisor." In her letter, "K.A.G." of Copperas Grove, Texas, said that she had a good marriage, but a problem threatened it: after nine years of having her hair chemically straightened, she wanted to let the perm grow out. But her man resisted. "My husband feels that I will become undesirable to him and has said that he might leave me if I do [let my perm grow out]. I'd hate to lose him or leave him because of this, but I dislike the trouble and illusion straightening my hair brings me. I long to be free of chemicals and I wish he would accept me 'naturally.'"

The "Ebony Advisor" conceded that the woman had the right to change her style but recommended that, since exercising her right would jeopardize her marriage, she should continue with the chemicals. The advisor reminded the reader that beauty is in the eye of the beholder, and told her that if her husband said, "Don't go changing," she should mind him. It's not much to pay to "keep the gleam in his eye gleaming."

SPLITTING HAIRS

On the one hand brothers have made a transition [to natural styles], and yet they don't expect the same of their women. They still want their women to be Asian women dipped in chocolate.

—Peggy Dillard Toone, Natural Hair Care Pioneer

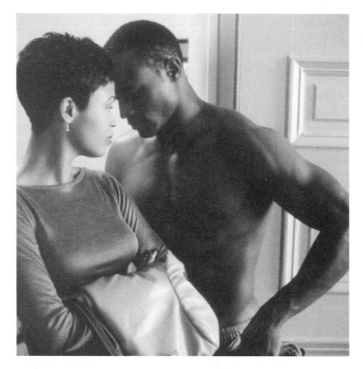

Taye Diggs and Nia Long feel that body heat in 1999's The Best Man.

PHOTOFEST

Although Diahann Carroll played a beleaguered, single mom in the 1974 film Claudine, *every hair on her head was in place. James Earl Jones's character was digging it.*

PHOTOFEST

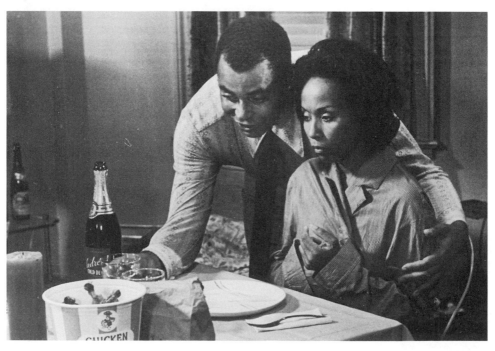

IF YOU LET ME MAKE LOVE TO YOU,
THEN WHY CAN'T I TOUCH YOUR HAIR?
Cherilyn "Liv" Wright

In 1970 Ronnie Dyson, the precocious black teenage star of the counterculture Broadway musical *Hair*, recorded the Top Forty hit "If You Let Me Make Love to You, Then Why Can't I Touch You?" While the irony and poignancy of the lyric might have been lost on some, at the time it struck this black college junior as profound.

It was from the dustbin of memory, then, that I heard the now-late Dyson singing in my ear as Angie, the twenty-something black receptionist at my client's office, told me that she had trained her boyfriend not to touch her hair while they were making love. I had complimented her on her freshly done, magazine-ready hairdo, which had been chemically straightened, tinted light brown, and augmented by straight, shoulder-length human hair that had been tightly woven to her scalp. Just brushing her forehead, and barely touching her eyebrow, was a flirtatious wisp of a curl.

"Can I touch it?" I asked.

"Sure," she said.

The wisp was as hard as a rock! "How did they get it to go like that?" I blurted.

"I dunno," she shrugged. "I guess they used gel or something, and then put me under the dryer to bake it in."

"Special occasion?"

"I'm going to see my boyfriend for the weekend."

"Well, what are you going to do about your hair when you and your boyfriend are doing 'the wild thing'?" I continued to probe. "Won't he think your hair is too stiff?"

"Oh, no, no, no, he knows he'd better not touch my hair!" she replied emphatically. "It costs me too much money. Oh, no, no, no, you have to train these men right away."

I couldn't believe my ears! Was it her tender age that caused her to place such a high priority on her hair? And didn't this hands-off-the-hair policy offend her boyfriend? Perplexed, I cornered an older black female associate for a sanity check.

"I'm worried about Angie," I said. "She's got a guy she's serious about, and she won't let him touch her hair when they make love! How does she expect to be really intimate with him?"

"Where have you been?" my colleague responded brutally. "There's nothing wrong with Angie. She's got a strategy that's working for her, and she's got plenty of company. You've obviously never talked to your girlfriends about what they do when they get together with their men. Black men do not expect to have their hands in our hair when we make love. Ask them."

She was right. I didn't have a clue. How many of my friends had given the hands-off message to their sex partners? And what did the menfolk have to say about all this? I picked up the phone and called one of my closest friends.

TRUDY'S EXTENSIONS

Trudy, a legal secretary, has been my friend since the fifth grade. We got our ears pierced about the same time, started menstruating about the same time, and debriefed one another after our "first time" with a boy. There isn't much we don't know about each other. Or so I thought.

"No, Mike doesn't touch my hair. I don't tell him not to in so many words, but I know he gets the point. The trick is to make your hair look touchable, but to make sure they don't actually touch it."

I was a maid of honor at Trudy's wedding ten years ago. Her husband, Mike, is a big lug of a guy who absolutely adores her. Long ago, I encouraged her to choose him over the other men she'd been dating. I told her that when they were both a hundred years old, and she forgot to take out her dentures before falling asleep, he would be the kind of guy to take them out for her and put them in a cup on the night table beside the bed.

"You have no idea what I went through to get a style that would work for me on our honeymoon," she said. "I wanted my hair to look free and playful when we were on the beach. But I wanted it to look elegant when we dressed for dinner on the ship. Remember how I had it done for the wedding?"

I confessed that I didn't. All I could remember was that the sweltering heat had ruined everyone's hairdo.

"I asked the beautician to give me some extensions because Mike and I were going on this honeymoon cruise and I didn't want to have to worry about my hair. I wanted to be able to use the pool and enjoy the beach when the ship stopped at one of the islands. I told her I wanted braids that would take me from the wedding ceremony to a sexy afternoon on the beach with my husband. She said she'd give me extensions that I could either pin up or wear long. For the wedding, she pinned the extensions way up on my head to give me height and a very regal look, remember?"

In the wedding pictures her hair is swept up into a Madame Pompadour-like tower, making Trudy, who normally stands five-foot-two, look almost as tall as her six-foot-four husband.

"The hairdresser also showed me how to remove the pins and wear it in a long style. I wanted to be able to fool around with Mike on the beach, make love with him in the water, and not have a problem. You know what I'm saying?"

I pictured Trudy as a bronze-toned cross between Bo Derek and Esther Williams, skipping across some Caribbean beach with Mike lumbering behind in hot pursuit.

"So the beautician braided extra hair into the extensions to make them a little thicker, and to hold them in place. If my hair got wet, no big deal, right? Well what she neglected to tell me was that when those extensions get wet, you're carrying another twenty pounds of weight on your head! And 100 percent human hair, when it's woven into heavy braids like that, doesn't dry for a real long time.

"So there I am that night dining with my husband at the captain's table, trying to sit up straight and keep my head from falling into my swordfish. It was a mess, girl!"

HARRIET'S WEAVE

I called Harriet next. Trudy and I used to hang out with her in high school. She was always one of our more glamorous friends. Harriet knows all the "in" places to get your hair done and always has the trendiest style.

She likes to think of herself as a seductress.

"I love the feel of a man's fingers massaging my scalp, but you can't let him do that when you have a weave," said Harriet when I put the question to her. "You want the intimacy, but you just can't. If the men like all this long hair, they need to be appreciative of what you've done to get it to look that way. But, don't get me wrong now, they don't need to know every little thing!"

"What do you mean when you say every little thing?" I ask.

"You know what I'm talking about. You have this fabulous weave, and he starts to run his fingers through it. But what it feels like to him, though, is that you have these tracks in your head! And then you hear him say, 'Oops.' And when you feel him slowly pulling his hands away, you know you've been found out! And you know what he's thinking. So then I start thinking about what he's thinking."

With all those imaginary voices in her head, I'm wondering if Harriet has ever had a real orgasm!

"When it comes to my hair," she says, pulling me back into the conversation, "I believe that some things are better left unsaid. My philosophy is to deal with the situation on a need-to-know basis only. If he's talking about marriage and giving me a ring, then okay, I'll take him backstage and show him how the hair routine was put together."

"You've really thought this whole thing out, haven't you?" I prompt her.

"Look, whatever it takes. My cousin Lossie's been married three years and still hasn't told her husband that that's not her real hair!"

MARK'S WIFE

It was time to get a male perspective on the situation, so I called Mark, a bona fide husband of more than twenty years. A suburban, Republican business owner, Mark is married to Jean, a public-sector administrator, who chemically relaxes her hair and never misses her semimonthly salon appointments. Mark and I have been friends for a long time and can talk about anything. I asked him about the hair rules in his household.

"The fellas always say that there are two things you can't get a black woman to do in bed: one is to perform oral sex and the other is to let you touch her hair. I'm very clear that I'm not supposed to touch my wife's hair."

"How do you feel about that?" I ask.

"I don't know, but I can tell you—and don't hate me for this, Cherilyn—that all black men basically want the same thing: light skin, light eyes, and long hair." (Don't hate me for this, Mark, but take a hike! Just because we can talk about anything, doesn't mean you should!)

"For some reason, though," he continued, "I've always been a little different. I prefer dark-brown-skinned women like my wife, but I've got to have the hair, see? And my wife knows it. She has beautiful hair, and it always looks great! So she can really play me, see? When it looks like I'm going to touch her hair, she'll say, 'C'mon, Mark, I just had my hair done, and I want it to last for a while. You want me to look nice for you, don't you?' So I leave her alone."

I'm curious now. Mark and his wife have four children, so I know that they have had a connubial liaison or two over the past couple of decades. "What does she do about her hair when the two of you finally get together?" I inquire.

"She puts on a scarf so her hair doesn't get messed up."

"All the time?"

"Yeah, mostly. Sometimes, if it's the day before her appointment with the hairdresser, or if we're on vacation, she'll make love without the scarf. It's almost like a concession from her, though."

"Is that all right with you?" I probe.

"Not really, but it's not worth it for me to make a big issue out of it. After twenty years of marriage, I've learned to pick my battles. If I'm asking her to give me all 999 positions in the *Kama Sutra,* I'm willing to settle for the stupid scarf."

I ask Mark how many scarves his wife has in her bedtime repertoire and if he knows what any of them look like. He says she has two, and yes, he kinda knows what they look like, but no, he can't exactly describe them to me.

I try to picture a romantic scene in Mark's household. I know that when couples make love (at least the way they show it on *All My Children),* there is a certain heightened emotional moment. The two lovers—lying side by side, gazing deeply into one another's eyes—pierce through those liquid windows of the soul to seduce each other with the "look." I ask Mark what he's thinking when he gazes at his wife during their concupiscent moment, and sees these scarves.

"It's funny," he says, "but I don't even notice the scarf. What I'm really looking at when I gaze into her face is its impeccable symmetry, the perfect brown depth of her skin, and her eyes locked into mine. My wife doesn't always want to make eye contact with me when we make love, but when she does, and when we really connect with each other, Lord, I'm a happy man! No, after all these years of marriage, I don't even see the scarf anymore. It's just always been there."

A neat, two-decade-long ménage-à-trois, I think to myself: Mark, his wife, and her scarf.

STEPHANIE'S HIGH-MAINTENANCE LOOK

My Generation X friend Stephanie, who has just turned thirty, has her own headwrap strategy. She has an exciting job in the entertainment industry in Los Angeles and spends her evenings after work at "listening parties" hosted by record producers and at screenings hosted by film companies. She's looking for a husband and would prefer a love connection with a man in her field. She tells me that because it is so "competitive" out there, any woman who is serious about her marriage-mission needs to be serious about looking good.

When I told her about Angie training her boyfriend not to touch her hair, Stephanie told me about her efforts to "break in" a new boyfriend. "I'd had my eye on this man for a long time, right? We kept running into one another at some of the parties I go to after work, and eventually we started to date. I'd already had him over for dinner, and this was going to be my first evening at his place. We hadn't been intimate yet, but I had the feeling that this might be the night. So I knew that everything had to be correct. Manicure. Pedicure. Massage. Waxing. And, of course, The Hair.

"It took me all day to get my hair the way I wanted it. I had to drive to the salon. Wait my turn. Shampoo. Condition. Trim. Set. Dry. Style. Drive home. That's eight hours. A whole day! So I knew that, no matter what happened at his house, it was going to be a don't-touch-my-hair evening. So, when he and I started to fool around in his living room and I told him not to touch my hair, he said, 'You've got to be kidding!' And, of course, it killed the whole mood."

"What happened then?" I asked.

"Nothing. We just sat and listened to music. I had brought some ice cream, so we ate that and watched a video."

"Was there an encore? I mean, did you see him again?"

"Yeah. We were basically all right with each other. So, the next time, I brought my do rag with me."

"The one with the magic powers?" I giggle because all black women have a faithful servant that holds our hair in place like nothing else.

"Yeah, that one. I've had it since college, and I took it in case I wanted to tie up my hair," she said, grinning from ear to ear. "But my date saw the do rag and broke out with 'What's that thing for?'

"I said, 'Never mind,' and put it away. It was funny though, because when I unwrapped the condom and started to put it on him, he said the same thing, 'What's that?' And I had to really tell him that if we were going to hang together, he was gonna have to wear his rain boots! I told him that I might be willing to compromise on the do rag, but definitely not on the boots."

AL'S WIFE

At sixty-two, Al is divorced from his wife of thirty years, and dates only the twenty-something Angies and Generation X Stephanies. "Women over forty want to talk," he explains, "especially the ones who went to college. But the younger ones? They'll sit and listen to a guy like me as long as I keep buying things for them."

I realize that with Al I have descended much lower on the food chain than I had intended. But I do want to hear what he has to say on the subject of hair and the art of making love. I know that Al's wife would have been part of the press 'n' curl, pre-chemical-straightener generation, and I ask him whether she'd had rules about not touching her hair.

"My stuck-up wife? Noooooo, you couldn't touch her hair!" He gestures wildly.

I ask whether he thinks this rule about hair is widespread and whether the younger women he dates let him touch their hair.

"No, I haven't had a problem with that, and I don't really think it's too widespread. Lemme see. Of the five hundred women I've slept with [Is he trying to impress someone?] only about five wouldn't let me touch their hair. Yeah, that's about right."

I'm preparing to build my statistical model from Al's sample (5 out of 500 is 1 percent). Then a pang of humility strikes, and Al begins to scale back his Wilt Chamberlain pretensions. "Well, maybe it was closer to four hundred. But I know it was definitely more than three hundred, 'cause one time I counted."

(If you say so, Al.)

He starts talking about his wife's hair again: "Nope. Could not touch it. She was so uptight about it that when we were lying there in the bed next to each other, she would actually ask me not to breathe so hard in her direction! Told me it would mess up her hair."

Of course! I totally understand where Al's wife is coming from. It's right there in any high school chemistry book. You can look it up. The chemical composition of human exhalation is CO_2 and H_2O, or carbon dioxide and water vapor. There is no scientific term, however, for the chemical reaction that occurs when water makes contact with African hair that's been pressed and curled. So, for generations, black women have settled for the prosaic expression, "My hair went back."

I wasn't sure where our hair went when it "went back" until I read a health and beauty book written in the mid-1970s by black supermodel Naomi Simms. She concludes her brief discourse on "The Heat Method of Hair Straightening" by informing the reader that, if the straightened hair is exposed to water, steam, or excessive humidity, it will return to its "original configuration."

So there it was. Al's wife was trying to keep the excessive humidity of her husband's breath from returning her hair to its original configuration! I asked Al what he said when she told him not to breathe on her. He grinned devilishly, as if enjoying some private joke. "I told her that if she'd just stop talking, and put her head down to a place where it could really do me some good, she wouldn't have to worry about my breathing on her hair."

LORNA'S HAIR ROLLERS

Unlike Al's wife, my friend Lorna is a black women who loves oral sex. She grew up during a time when a teenage girl was able to remain "technically" a virgin while giving blow jobs like crazy at the drive-in movie. She's been married to Craig since she was in her early twenties. They are in their forties now and haven't lost any of their heat.

"I don't know where that character came from," said all-the-way-from-New Orleans Lorna, after I told her Al's story, "but these men complain even when you do go down there to try to make them feel good."

Lorna has slept in hair rollers every night since she was in high school, and her good-natured husband, Craig, has accustomed himself to conjugal bliss with a human porcupine. "He calls it my 'bedroom furniture,'" Lorna says, sucking her teeth and mocking offense. She's referring to her inventory of curling implements that reads like a quarter-century of discount hair-care catalogs: wire mesh rollers, large juice cans, small juice cans, sponge curlers, metal rollers, magnetic rollers, pastel-colored plastic rollers in graduated sizes, rollers with Velcro, rollers that twist, rollers that bend in half, rollers with teeth. And Craig's privates have had their share of violent encounters with them all.

"I try to be real careful," Lorna insisted, "but it seems like somehow something's always happening. Craig keeps asking me why all the things I put on my head have such a sharp edge, but they really don't. It just depends on how you move around."

For years, Craig's nemesis was the pink plastic pin made by the Goody Company to hold the wire mesh rollers in place. "He was always fussing with me about how these little pink pins kept getting stuck in his creases. I had no idea what he was talking about! What kinda creases? All I know is that when I was down there foolin' around, these little pins seemed like they always wanna fall out. Shoot, here I was gettin' him off! I know he didn't hardly think I was gonna let him go limp on me to try and track down some pins to see where they went."

YVONNE'S WIG

Yvonne never rolls her hair. She's a wig person. And now that I think about it, I may never have seen her real hair. Yvonne is the kind of woman who sends her wigs out for shampooing as often as she sends her silk blouses to the dry cleaners. I asked her about her lovemaking strategy.

"You must never let them touch the Wendy," Yvonne said, preening.

"What's the Wendy?" I asked.

"Your Wendy, girl! Your hair. I always name my wigs Wendy. Every generation of black women has had their Wendy, and, like American Express, you don't leave home without her. Wendy used to be a fall, a long braid, a chignon, a wig, even (Lord have mercy) an Afro wig! Today, Wendy can be a weave, extensions, locks."

I never knew Yvonne to be an armchair philosopher, but I was compelled by her thesis.

"A black girl learns very early that she is either a 'hair-have' or a 'hair-have-not.' And when your hair doesn't grow quickly, you have to attract the man you want by any means necessary. You have to learn to hold your own because you're competing with all the other girls—black ones, white ones, Asian ones, Spanish ones, Native American ones—who have hair."

This is the second time in my little survey that someone has mentioned competition with other women as one of her motivating concerns.

"So when I was at the Rhythm 'n' Blues Foundation Awards last winter, I noticed that everybody was wearing a Wendy, and said to myself, 'This is my crowd.' Yeah, this was the wig crowd. We grew up knowing that that wasn't Tina Turner's real hair, or puh-leese, Diana Ross's! These women have been our models since we were kids. They're stars. And when you're wearing your Wendy, you're a star, too. I know I feel like one. You tell yourself, my hair is my little secret. And if a woman is good in bed and puts a freak on for her man, he won't even think about touching her hair!"

Indeed, Yvonne had earned somewhat of a reputation for putting her legendary "freak" on a roster of men that read like the Rhythm 'n' Blues Hall of Fame. As a teenager in Harlem, she was a regular visitor backstage at the Apollo Theatre, where she was permitted to stand in the wings while the major attractions performed. At first her innocent flirtations led to teen fantasies that Smokey Robinson and David Ruffin were singing their love songs just for her. By the time she was in her early twenties, however, she had become a regular in the stars' dressing rooms and in their hotel suites. After the midnight show, wearing Wendy like a crown, Yvonne would strut out the stage door, escorted by her conquest du jour, and duck into one of the black limousines parked along West 126th Street.

"When I used to make bubble baths for a romantic evening, especially when my date wanted to relax in the tub after the last show, I'd be sure to hold Wendy just above the water line—like an invisible barrier—to keep her dry. With both of us having such a good time, why would he need to touch the Wendy? Really. Hey, I could freak in a tub full of water, and not wet a single strand! I'd be thinking that whoever used to own this hair can't possibly be having as much fun as I am!"

WALTER'S MORNING AFTER

The latter-day Wendy, the weave, seems not to have survived the marathon night my friend Walter spent with his date, Janet. Walter is the garden-variety "nice guy" who is always complaining that he can't find a "nice lady." He's an easygoing, laid-back type who says that he's looking for a steady companion. He thought that Janet was the one.

"I know that some women are funny about their hair. But this one time when Janet and I were really getting into it, she stopped cold and told me that if I messed up her hair, I'd have to pay for it. I thought she was joking, and I tried to say something smart like: 'Oh, so now it's dinner, a movie and a trip to the hair salon!' She didn't laugh, though; she was serious. I didn't want to be the one to ruin the whole night, so I went with the flow and said, 'Okay, baby, no problem.'"

I asked Walter how he felt when Janet told him that he'd have to pay for her hair. Frankly, I was surprised that he had been caught off guard by her straightforward request for reimbursement. I'd have thought that, at this stage in their relationship, she would have already "trained" him, or they would have somehow handled the issue. Walter told me that by the time Janet presented her ultimatum, he was too aroused to negotiate better terms for himself, and he was prepared to concede whatever was necessary to score the touchdown.

"It was great, though," Walter mused, savoring the memory. "We were into each other all night long, having a real good time. But when we woke up the next morning, I felt something funny on the sheet. I reached underneath my behind, and there was all this hair! Everywhere! All over the bed, all over the floor. Wads of it! I looked at her and she looked at me, and we both started laughing. Next thing I know we're crawling around on all fours scooping up hair. I never felt so stupid in my whole life. Here I was picking up all this hair, and putting it in a pile on my dresser! So, I looked at her, and asked her what she wanted to do with it."

She went ballistic:

"What do I want to do with it? No, no. It's not what I want to do with it, it's what I'm going to do with it. I'm going to pack it up and take it to my hairdresser so she can sew it back on my head. What did you think I wanted to do with it?"

"I was just asking, baby."

"I hope you have a shopping bag? You don't think I'm going to walk down the street with my hands full of hair, do you?"

Walter told me that, at that moment, the whole scene began to feel like punishment for some bad thing he had done a very long time ago.

"So, in my bare feet, I go into the kitchen to look for a large bag. The floor's cold. I'm feeling guilty. I just want to pay her the money and go back to bed. I can't find a shopping bag but I figure that if I can give her one of my old shirts to use as a makeshift bag, I can calm her down. I go back to the bedroom to find a shirt. We wrap the wads of hair in the shirt, and tie the shirttail and sleeves together."

Even now, as Walter tells me the story about the wads of hair, it's still hard for him not to laugh. What was not so funny for Walter, however, was the conversation he had with Janet about paying for her hair. He's an honorable guy, and meant it when he promised to pay for it.

"How much do you need, Janet?"

"Two hundred dollars."

"You're joking."

"No, I'm not. This is 100 percent human hair. Sterilized. This is quality, Walter!"

Walter told me that he believed this was God's way of telling him something. But he wasn't sure exactly what. Two hundred dollars, he said, is a little less than the annual premium for his fire insurance. It was one hundred fifty gallons of gas for his car. One hundred Big Macs. A premium ticket to the NBA playoffs. A couple of shares of Microsoft stock.

"But two hundred dollars to sew on some hair?" Walter asks me rhetorically. "That's ridiculous. I wouldn't care if it was hair from Her Majesty the Queen that had been sterilized in holy water drawn from the sacred fountains of St. Peter's Basilica in Rome!"

I asked Walter what he said to Janet after she told him how much it cost.

"I said, 'Okay, baby, no problem.' But I thought to myself, This is the last time I'm gonna pay to sew some hair into somebody's head. From now on when I meet a woman I think I could get interested in, I'm gonna say, 'Hi, my name is Walter. Excuse me, but do you mind my asking if that's your real hair?'"

ARLENE'S CHOREOGRAPHY

My friend Arlene told me that she learned her lesson about hair weaves the same way Janet did—the hard way. She teaches business English at a junior college, and always had a gift for styling her hair. Over the fifteen years that we've been friends, her hairstyles have ranged from natural to relaxed to cornrows to weaves. She says she's through with weaves forever but still likes to protect her hairstyle when she does the wild thing.

"What I notice more than anything about my lovemaking is that, no matter what kind of style I have, I always keep my eyes open to make sure that my partner isn't coming for my head! I never let my head get in the way of the action."

I ask Arlene what it feels like to be a sentry-on-duty while she's making love. It seems impossible to enjoy yourself while maintaining that kind of vigilance over your partner's moves.

"It's not a problem, really," Arlene explains. "You learn to protect your hair by moving your neck back and forth, and swinging your head from side to side to avoid contact. You stay on top, and learn to master the superior position, that's all."

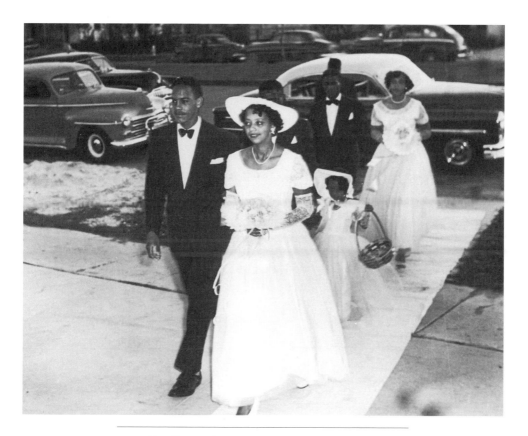

Heading to the altar with freshly minted curls.

ROBERT PERRY III, ALLFORD TROTMAN

"I see." I nod affirmatively with each of her well-orchestrated countermoves and wonder whether Arlene is a participant or an observer in this activity.

"You mount and use your moves in a way that keeps the mood going," she continues. "Oh yeah, you really get into it. You're on top swinging around and around, and he ain't hardly thinking about touching your hair!"

℮ LOVE POTIONS 1-4 ℮

Collected by Constance Johnson

Ain't no reason to be lonely when you can draw a man right to you with these tried and true Love Drawing Spells. They come from the same folks who worked High John the Conquerer and invented seven varieties of mojo:

1. Take a strand of his hair and put it in the Bible. After five days, take it out and put it in a perfume bottle. He will fall madly in love with you. (Now, after you get him, don't do nothing silly like taking the hair out of the perfume bottle!)

2. Take two strands of hair from the man you be wanting and place each hair in the heel of each of your shoes. Now wear them for nine days. The hair will continue to grow, and just as it do, so will his love for you.

3. Love relations been going poor lately? Take a pair of his old shoes and put some of your hair in 'em and wear 'em. That'll bring him on back to you. Remember now, the spell only last if you continue to wear the shoes. Take away the shoes or the hair from the shoes, he gone leave you again, so be careful.

4. This one is a little trickier. It require that you know someone that got a mole on they head, and the mole gotta have hair growing out of it. Now what you do is to take some graveyard dirt and mix it with some hair from that mole. Now put it all in a little sack and carry it in your pocket. This also is a good luck charm. Adding a dime in with the graveyard dirt and a lock of a hair (from a woman if your intended is a woman, the opposite if your love object is a man). This will also make the other person want you.

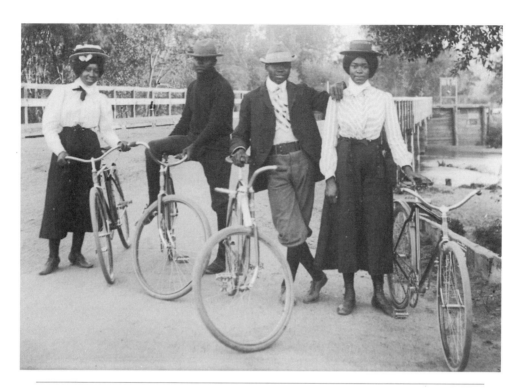

Rolling on the River, 1900s. The hats fit nicely over the women's molded hair as they stood on a river's edge in Denver, but what happened when they got their wheels in motion?

COLORADO HISTORICAL SOCIETY

BATTLE OF THE WIGS
George C. Wolfe

In *The Colored Museum*, playwright George C. Wolfe personified the "good hair/bad hair" dialectic by pitting an Afro wig named Janine against a straight-haired wig named LaWanda, in an argument about which should be worn by a bald-headed woman. The woman, whose hair is a chemical casualty, is preparing for an important date with her boyfriend and needs all the help she can get.

JANINE: What do mean you ain't made up your mind! After all that fool has put you through, you gonna need all the attitude you can get and there is nothing like attitude and a healthy head of kinks to make his shit shrivel like it should!

That's right! When you wearin' me, you lettin' him know he ain't gonna get no sweet-talkin', comb-through-your-love without some serious resistance. No-no! The kink of my head is like the kink of your heart, and neither is about to be hot-pressed into surrender.

LAWANDA: That shit is so tired. The last time attitude worked on anybody was 1968. Janine, girl, you need to get over it and get on with it. (Turning to the Woman.) And you need to give the nigga a good-bye he will never forget.

I say give him hysteria! Give him emotion! Give him rage! And there is nothing like a toss of the tresses to make your emotional outburst shine with emotional flair.

You can toss me back, shake me from side to side, all while screaming, I want you out of my life forever!!!

JANINE: Miss hunny, please! She don't need no Barbie doll dipped in chocolate telling her what to do. She needs a head of hair that's coming from a fo' real place.

LAWANDA: Don't you dare talk about nobody coming from a "fo' real place," Miss Made-in-Taiwan!

ONLY YOU

Among the Maroons of South America's Suriname, one popular hairdo of the past was known as "come this evening" or "husband and wife"; a woman would create the pattern of intertwined braids only for a man she loved.

—Sally and Richard Price, *Afro-American Arts of the Suriname Rain Forest*

"When I was in high school, I used to get girls by telling them, 'Come over to my house: I'll mess your hair up and fix it back again.'"

—Fred Parnell, Hairdresser, Brooklyn

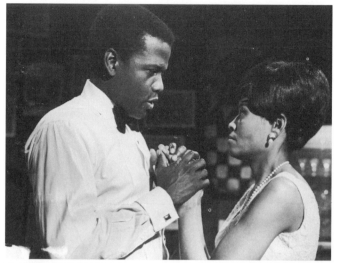

Abbey Lincoln (with Sidney Poitier) covered her Afro with a wig to play a maid in 1968's For Love of Ivy.

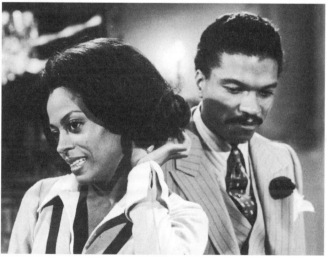

Success is nothing without someone to share it with: Diana Ross and Billy Dee Williams share the spotlight in the 1972 film Lady Sings the Blues.

WHITE BOYFRIEND
Evangeline Wheeler

If he hadn't rushed me, I would have packed my favorite curling iron, the medium-size silver one with the black handle. It was too early in the morning to be running around looking for things. I was still too drowsy and irritable, moments after he got me out of a toasty bed on a chilly dawn. I didn't need to be hurried.

We had planned a three-hour drive along the coast and a leisurely day at the ocean. Though I had looked forward to it the night before, by morning I had turned grumpy. So when he asked me at the blush of daybreak if I wanted to get dinner and a hotel room later that evening, I agreed, but wasn't clearheaded enough to pack a bag for the evening. I grabbed only a dress, a slip, some soft sandals, and some lipstick, and scurried behind him through the front door. When we had driven about a mile from the apartment, I remembered the curling iron, but he refused to go back for it, and we argued.

It was the hair argument all over again. I couldn't count the number of times we'd had this discussion during our years together, but it was probably at least once a week. He was always curious about things like why African Americans didn't go to Woody Allen films, and what made our skin ashy, which he called "chalky." It was a black thing, and he was white. When the conversation turned to hair differences, he was so perplexed by what we sisters did to ours. "Why can't you just wash it and let the sun dry it?" he'd ask.

He likened his hair to a dirt attractant, a repository of all the vehicle exhaust, air pollution, cigarette smoke, and ventilator dust that he encountered daily as he romped around San Francisco, where he lived. It disgusted him that I put a substance such as pomade that attracted dirt into my hair, and then didn't wash it out for several days. Obviously, he didn't understand black hair.

"I can't get into bed at night without showering and washing my hair," he'd say, trying to make me feel dirty. "How can you go all week without a shampoo when you know all this greasy dirt is getting on your pillows and sheets at night?"

To him, my use of a shower cap was contrary to cleanliness. "You step into a shower to wash up all over," he reasoned, "so it's stupid to cover up some of your dirty parts with plastic."

As I would go on the defensive, explaining why I was dependent on the curling iron, or why my roots had a different texture from the hair on top, or why humidity is such a terribly destructive force, his message was seeping in. I heard him, I really heard him, and I felt the shame of what I was doing to myself. Why couldn't I simply step out into the world with my hair the way it was?

EXCERPT FROM *SONG OF SOLOMON*
Toni Morrison

In a small town in Michigan in the early 1960s, Hagar, a young woman from an all-female family of social outcasts, desperately loves her well-to-do cousin, Macon ("Milkman") Dead. If she can make herself beautiful, she thinks, then maybe he will love her. So she sets off on a shopping spree.

She bought a Playtex garter belt, I. Miller No Color hose, Fruit of the Loom panties, and two nylon slips—one white, one pink—one pair Joyce Fancy Free and one of Con Brio ("Thank heaven for little Joyce heels"). She carried an armful of skirts and an Evan-Picone two-piece number into the fitting room. Her little yellow dress that buttoned all the way down lay on the floor as she slipped a skirt over her head and shoulders, down to her waist. But the placket would not close. She sucked in her stomach and pulled the fabric as far as possible, but the teeth of the zipper would not join. A light sheen broke out on her forehead as she huffed and puffed. She was convinced that her whole life depended on whether or not those aluminum teeth would meet. The nail of her forefinger split and the balls of her thumbs ached as she struggled with the placket. Dampness became sweat, and her breath came in gasps. She was about to weep when the saleswoman poked her head through the curtain and said brightly, "How are you doing?" But when she saw Hagar's gnarled and frightened face, the smile froze.

"Oh, my," she said, and reached for the tag hanging from the skirt's waist. "This is a five. Don't force it. You need, oh, a nine or eleven, I should think. Please. Don't force it. Let me see if I have that size."

She waited until Hager let the plaid skirt fall down to her ankles before disappearing. Hagar easily drew on the skirt the woman brought back, and without further search, said she would take it and the little two-piece Evan-Picone.

She bought a white blouse next and a nightgown—fawn trimmed in sea foam. Now all she needed was makeup.

The cosmetics department enfolded her in perfume, and she read hungrily the labels and the promise. Myrurgia for primeval woman who creates for him a world of tender privacy where the only occupant is you, mixed with Nina Ricci's L'Air du Temps. Yardley's Flair with Tuvaché's Nectaroma and D'Orsay's Intoxication. Robert Piguet's Fracas, and Calypso and Visa and Bandit. Houbigant's Chantilly. Caron's Fleurs de Rocaille and Bellodgia. Hagar breathed deeply the sweet air that hung over the glass counters. Like a smiling sleepwalker she circled. Round and round the diamond-clear counters covered with bottles, wafer-thin disks, round boxes, tubes, and phials. Lipsticks in soft white hands darted out of the sheaths like the shiny red penises of puppies. Peachy powders and milky lotions were grouped in front of poster after cardboard poster of gorgeous grinning faces. Faces in ecstasy. Faces somber with achieved seduction. Hagar believed she could spend her life there among the cut glass, shimmering in peaches and cream, in satin. In opulence. In luxe. In love.

It was five-thirty when Hagar left the store with two shopping bags full of smaller bags gripped in her hands. And she didn't put them down until she reached Lilly's Beauty Parlor.

"No more heads, honey," Lilly looked up from the sink as Hagar came in.

Hagar stared. "I have to get my hair done. I have to hurry," she said.

Lilly looked over at Marcelline. It was Marcelline who kept the shop prosperous. She was younger, more recently trained, and could do a light press that lasted. Lilly was still using red hot irons and an ounce of oil on every head. Her customers were loyal but dissatisfied. Now she spoke to Marcelline, "Can you take her? I can't, I know."

Marcelline peered deeply into her customer's scalp. "Hadn't planned on any late work. I got two more coming. This is my eighth today."

No one spoke. Hagar stared.

"Well," said Marcelline. "Since it's you, come on back at eight-thirty. But don't expect nothing fancy."

"I'm surprised by you," Lilly chuckled when Hagar left. "You just sent two people away."

"Yeah, well, I don't feel like it, but I don't want any trouble with that girl Hagar. No telling what she might do. She jump that cousin of hers, no telling what she might do to me."

"That the one going with Macon Dead's boy?" Lilly's customer lifted her head away from the sink.

"That's her. Ought to be shamed, the two of them. Cousins."

"Must not be working out if she's trying to kill him."

"I thought he left town."

"Wouldn't you?"

"Well, I know I don't want to truck with her. Not me."

"She don't bother nobody but him."

"Well, Pilate, then. Pilate know I turned her down, she wouldn't like it. They spoil that child something awful."

"Didn't you order that fish from next door?"

"All that hair. I hope she don't expect nothing fancy."

"Call him up again. I'm getting hungry."

"Be just like her. No appointment. No nothing. Come in here all late and wrong and want something fancy."

She probably meant to wait somewhere. Or go home and return to Lilly's at eight-thirty. Yet the momentum of the thing held her—it was all of a piece. From the moment she looked into the mirror in the little pink compact she could not stop. It was as though she held her breath and could not let it go until the energy and busyness culminated in a beauty that would dazzle him. That was why, when she left Lilly's, she looked neither right nor left but walked on and on, oblivious of other people, street lights, automobiles, and a thunderous sky. She was thoroughly soaked before she realized it was raining and then only because one of the shopping bags split. When she looked down her Evan-Picone white-with-a-band-of-color skirt was lying in a neat half fold on the shoulder of the road, and she was far far from home. She put down both bags, picked the skirt up and brushed away the crumbs of gravel that stuck to it. Quickly she refolded it, but when she tried to tuck it back in the shopping bag, the bag collapsed altogether. Rain soaked her hair and poured down her neck as she stooped to repair the damage. She pulled out the box of Con Brios, a smaller package of Van Raalte gloves, and another containing her fawn-trimmed-in-sea-foam shortie nightgown. These she stuffed into the other bag. Retracing her steps, she found herself unable to carry the heavier bag in one hand, so she hoisted it up on her stomach and hugged it with both arms. She had gone hardly ten yards when the bottom fell out of it. Hagar tripped on Jungle Red (Sculptura) and Youth Blend, and to her great dismay, saw her box of Sunny Glow toppling into a puddle. She collected Jungle Red and Youth Blend safely, but Sunny Glow, which had tipped completely over and lost its protective disk, exploded in light peach puffs under the weight of the raindrops. Hagar scraped up as much of it as she could and pressed the wilted cellophane disk back into the box.

Twice before she got to Darling Street she had to stop to retrieve her purchases from the ground. Finally she stood in Pilate's doorway, limp, wet, and confused, clutching her bundles in whatever way she could. Reba was so relieved to see her that she grabbed her, knocking Chantilly and Bandit to the floor. Hagar stiffened and pulled away from her mother.

"I have to hurry," she whispered. "I have to hurry."

Loafers sluicing, hair dripping, holding her purchases in her arms, she made it into her bedroom and shut the door. Pilate and Reba made no move to follow her.

Hagar stripped herself naked there, and without taking time to dry her face or hair or feet, she dressed herself up in the white-with-a-band-of-color skirt and matching bolero, the Maidenform brassiere, the Fruit of the Loom panties, the no color hose, the Playtex garter belt and the Joyce Con Brios. Then she sat down to attend to her face. She drew charcoal gray for the young round eye through her brows, after which she rubbed Mango Tango on her cheeks. Then she patted Sunny Glow all over her face. Mango Tango disappeared under it and she had to put it on again. She pushed out her lips and spread Jungle Red over them. She put baby clear sky light to outwit the day light on her eyelids and touched Bandit to her throat, earlobes, and wrists. Finally she poured a little Youth Blend into her palm and smoothed it over her face.

At last she opened the door and presented herself to Pilate and Reba. And it was in their eyes that she saw what she had not seen before in the mirror: the wet ripped hose, the soiled white dress, the sticky, lumpy face powder, the streaked rouge, and the wild wet shoals of hair. All this she saw in their eyes, and the sight filled her own with water warmer and much older than the rain. Water that lasted for hours, until the fever came, and then it stopped. The fever dried her eyes up as well as her mouth.

She lay in her little Goldilocks'-choice bed, her eyes sand dry and as quiet as glass. Pilate and Reba, seated beside the bed, bent over her like two divi-divi trees beaten forward by a wind always blowing from the same direction. Like the trees, they offered her all they had: love murmurs and a protective shade.

"Mama." Hagar floated up into an even higher fever.

"Hmmm?"

"Why don't he like my hair?"

"Who, baby? Who don't like your hair?"

"Milkman."

"Milkman does too like your hair," said Reba.

"No. He don't. But I can't figure out why. Why he never liked my hair."

"Of course he likes it. How can he not like it?" asked Pilate.

"He likes silky hair." Hagar was murmuring so low they had to bend down to hear her.

"Silky hair? Milkman?"

"He don't like mine."

"Hush, Hagar."

"Silky hair the color of a penny."

"Don't talk, baby."

"Curly, wavy, silky hair. He don't like mine."

Pilate put her hand on Hagar's head and trailed her fingers through her granddaughter's soft damp wool. "How can he not love your hair? It's the same hair that grows out of his armpits. The same hair that crawls up out his crotch on up his stomach. All over his chest. The very same. It grows out of his nose, over his lips, and if he ever lost his razor it would grow all over his face. It's all over his head, Hagar. It's his hair too. He got to love it."

"He don't love it at all. He hates it."

"No he don't. He don't know what he loves, but he'll come around, honey, one of these days. How can he love himself and hate your hair?"

"He loves silky hair."

"Hush, Hagar."

"Penny-colored hair."

"Please, honey."

"And lemon-colored skin."

"Shhh."

"And gray-blue eyes."

"Hush now, hush."

"And thin nose."

"Hush, girl, hush."

"He's never going to like my hair."

"Hush. Hush. Hush, girl, hush."

TRADITIONAL BLUES LYRIC

She's a kinky headed woman
And she keeps a combin' it all the time.
She's a kinky headed woman
And she keeps a combin' it all the time
I can't stand nothing she done,
She keeps good lookin' women on my mind.

DEKAR'S TOUCH
Pamela Johnson

For twenty years Dekar Lawson has stroked black women's hair, admired their beauty, and lent an empathetic ear to their stories. I first met him a few years back when I needed my ends trimmed. At the time, he was working in Harlem at Turning Heads, one of the nation's first natural hair-care shops.

A thin, attractive man with angular features, Dekar, forty, is a charmer. His manner—catching my eye and gently stroking my hair—was so seductive that I went home and wrote a short story (not knowing the spelling of his first name) called "The Wives of Dakar." For a hot moment, I wondered if he was really sparking me. Then I decoded it: His way was to make women feel wanted, special, beautiful under his touch. I figured he flirted with everybody, and that he'd cultivated a harem of customers, swirling around him, eager for their weekly fix. Some, I imagined, had no one else in their lives to touch them but Dekar.

The next time I went back for a trim, easily a year later, Dekar had moved on. Still, I remained curious about him. Then one day I was talking to a friend and, oddly enough, Dekar's name came up in the conversation. He and Dekar were related. I got the number and called. Once again I needed a trim, but more than that, I wanted to hear a male stylist's insights about women.

Dekar met me at the downstairs door, wearing a black-and-white-striped sweater, black slacks, and stylish Italian loafers, and escorted me up to his second-floor shop, Dekar Salon. I liked its exposed brick walls, smart black-and-

HEADS IN HARMONY

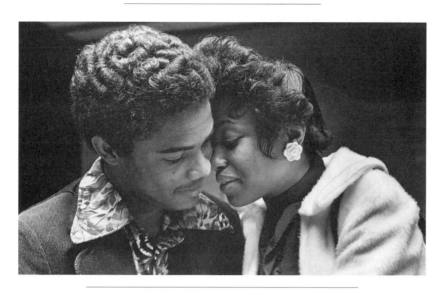

A couple cuddle in a club in Fort Wayne, Indiana, ca. 1970.

PETER TURNLEY/CORBIS

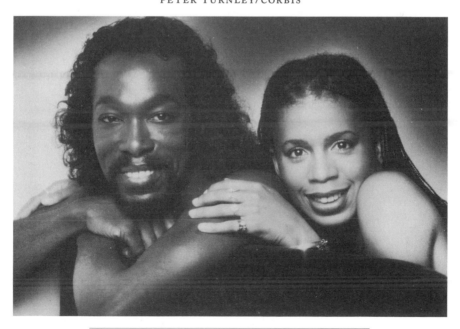

Nick ("Is It Still Good to You?") Ashford and Valerie Simpson.

PHOTOFEST

white tiles, and floor-to-ceiling glass windows, which look out on a cluster of boutiques on Lexington Avenue on Manhattan's Upper East Side. Dekar and I sat in opposing chairs, and then he snipped my ends, telling me what I'd come to hear. . . .

My clientele is mostly black women. But about 10 percent of my clientele is European American. I've got a couple of Spanish girls, and a couple of Jewish ladies who come in to get relaxers. I've got a few men, a couple of them are Spanish; they get texturizers because they have that wavy, nappy hair, and they want to smooth it out.

My clients don't usually confide in me, I'm more observant. You learn that with professional women, you don't ask them questions. I think it's because of the environment they work in; there they have to constantly watch their back and that [kind of caution] spills over into other relationships. But you can tell when they're kind of edgy; you can tell something's happening in their lives. Women who are blue collar, they'll talk to you. But I think in having this salon, which is more private [than the places I used to work], I have more intense conversations here. . . .

I love details, I love gossip, but I don't pry. Besides, some of the stuff they tell you hurts. They may be getting divorced or the husband or boyfriend is acting up. It hurts to see someone not treating them right.

Sometimes things can get really emotional. During one period, when I worked in another shop, every Friday for about six months, at least one of my clients cried. My coworkers looked at me like, 'What are you doing to them?' I said I don't know. I thought something was wrong with me. I'd be talking to somebody and say something that hit them, maybe I'm massaging their scalp, and suddenly they were in tears.

I think sometimes people hold it all in and then get in a situation where they can relax and somebody's stroking their head, and they start to think about [the incident that disturbed them] again. . . . I've seen people really boo-hoo. Me, I'm very discreet, I just go get the tissue, turn them away from the mirror, and stand in front of them. I'm thinking, After this, I'm going to need a drink, because I don't like to see people cry.

SOME LIKE IT SWEET

I notice that women enjoy being fawned over. I guess we all do. I try to keep that in mind, and I try to go places where they do that for me, so I remember how good it feels. When I was younger I would tell my assistants that I was going to act annoyed

when they interrupted me, like "Can't you see I'm busy taking care of this very impor-
tant person?" But I stopped doing that; it was corny. Still it's true: I don't like to be in-
terrupted; when I'm doing you, I'm just doing you. I don't like to be all over the place. If
you want me to tell you some jokes about me, to take your mind off your world and just
put it in my little frivolous one, fine. Or you can talk and I can listen, I like to listen.
What I don't like is when there's tension around here because one woman thinks I'm
paying another woman more attention than I'm paying her. Some people want all your
attention. Bottom line is, I'm just doing a service.

I do flirt though. But you can't flirt with really young women. They think you're
serious. I'm like nah, I ain't serious—I'm flirting. I didn't call you at home, did I? But
married women or older ladies, they know, and they flirt right back, because it's all
within a safe confine. Some people are waiting for you to make the next move, but it's
really in a box; it doesn't move any further than that. I don't flirt as much as I used to.
People can confuse things. The way I look at women, and I do like looking at women—
it can bring out certain emotions, I appreciate natural beauty and they can see that I
like it, I'm not joking around about that, and some women are really beautiful.

Some women use their beauty to get what they want. I tell them you better get
something upstairs because if you're walking down the street and you fall and break your
face, and you ain't getting paid, you're screwed. That's a really competitive world out
there—people who play people by using their looks to get what they need. You're gonna
get hurt in that game, because you play with a lot of guys who've got it like that. You're
just a number. They can spend $500 on you a night; that's no money to them. You think
you have the upper hand because he's spending money on you or giving you things, but
he's got a couple of girls, and you're nothing to him. When you figure that out, it hurts.

BLACK WOMEN AND WHITE WOMEN

White women feel freer to say, "I want to look sexy. Make my hair sexy." Black
women don't say that; they just say, "Make me look beautiful." White women use color
as much as black women use relaxers. But they don't have as many options as black
women. All they have is cut and color—the perm thing for them went out of style.
Black women have got it all over them. There's nothing they can't do: wear it straight
like them, wear it nappy, pin it up, roller set it, achieve all these different textures. It
can be really short and natural or really short and permed. Black women can use color.
They can get a lot of different looks, just by twisting the hair differently.

Still, some black women really hate their hair. They go from salon to salon, trying to get it to do something it's not ever going to do. My opinion comes after I put my hands in your hair. I say, "This is what your hair says it likes to do. If you follow it, you'll be happy with the least amount of struggle." The more you make your hair do something it doesn't want to, the more you've got to work. It's best when someone comes to me and says, "Make my hair look better," because then I can just do what it takes.

Most black women think white women got it easy; I personally think white people got more issues. They try to be more Anglo. They could be Polish, Italian, Greek, but they're trying to have a white Anglo-Saxon Protestant look. White women love blond because it's the color of youth, the color their hair was when they were five or ten. A lot of black people like Jada Pinkett Smith and RuPaul just use blond hair to have fun. They're not trying to be white. Neither are most black women who straighten their hair. For some black women, that's all they know; they've had their hair straightened since they were twelve. We're on that second generation of women who didn't grow up braiding their hair. They're eighteen, nineteen years old, and they can't braid or cornrow. They're not even familiar with their hair in its unpermed state. Some of them let the perm grow out for the first time as adults and go, "Wow, this is what it is? Give me the perm."

KEEPING IT ALL COORDINATED

The most I can do at once is three or four people. If I'm running behind, I call as many people as I can ahead of time and say, "Take your time because I'm not moving that fast today." The key to being able to take care of other people is to take care of your own personal needs before you come to work. If you don't take care of your needs, it's hard to be there for somebody else, 'cause you're trying to get soothed, too.

Mostly I listen to my clients, but I'll also talk about myself. Some people like that sharing; it's all frivolous for me. I'll talk about something that happened to me. My daughter is definitely a topic; she hates that, though. But women like to hear about what I go through as a single parent. Also, anytime I have a big decision to make, I ask everybody's opinion all week long, and then I make my decision. One time I did it after the fact, though. I had bought my daughter this crazily stupidly expensive Gucci bag. It was a purse she could have at eighteen years old, twenty years old, twenty-five years old. It was a special design they did, and it was on sale. It was still expensive. I didn't know that purses cost that much money.

So anyway, after I bought it, I took a survey with my clients. Half the women said, "You're foolish"; the other half were like, "See, your daughter's going to know that when some guy comes up to her, he's got to offer her the best because her father set the standard." The majority of the women who told me that were very confident. They don't take mess from nobody. A guy can't roll up on those women and say, "Oh, I'll let you ride in my Mercedes." They'd be like, "What does that mean? It might not even be yours."

What I learned was that a woman who is not treated really special as a girl works through that her whole life. And there are so many guys out there that know her number and they use it. It makes women mistrustful. So I think my daughter knows now that a guy's got to come with the best. He's got to come with some smarts, some grace, some charm, some sincerity. He's gotta come like that.

ON DATING CLIENTS

I've dated a few clients. Two of them turned into long-term relationships, and we're still best friends. Except for one person, I'm still friends with everybody. I still do their hair. Some got married, some are in relationships, but we can still hang out. I don't like to date clients anymore, though, because if you happen to break up, she's out of here, and her friends go with her. It doesn't matter what happened. It doesn't matter how good you did their hair, they'll stand by their girl.

There was this one lady who was gone for a while for another reason. When she came back, she was talking to me about coloring her hair. She was very particular. She asked a lot of questions, like, What is this you're using? I didn't catch it right away. But then I noticed that her hair had gone from curly to straight—and also that she had never asked me these kinds of questions before. Then it occurred to me that she was undergoing some kind of medical treatment.

You have to be really sensitive to people, because they could start asking you all these questions, and you could start getting defensive and annoyed. They may not want you to know what's going on with them. Or they may not be sure that you'll be sensitive to it. For some people, I've actually gone to the hospital to do their hair. Usually you're just cutting it off.

When my best friend died, I did her hair for the funeral. She was only thirty, and I didn't know she was that sick. I don't know whether it was cancer or what; she didn't want people to know. Doing hair under those circumstances is a special skill. The hair doesn't move the same. Death—it's a complete thing. It really touched me. It's very emotional. She was so cold, so cold. My hands were cold working on her. I tell you, enjoy life.

A HAIR-FREE FUTURE

I used to do my [four] sisters' hair when they came home for Christmas. Now they don't even ask me because they know I'm tired. On holidays, my usual position, before and after dinner, is asleep on the couch. So far I haven't had any health problems, but I have [hairstylist] friends who do. Their veins have fallen [in their legs] or their back gives out, because you're always working in a bent position, that's why I'm sitting in this chair like this. (He leans back against the chair with his feet up.) I require one day a week when I do nothing. Usually it's Sunday after church. I don't know how people do it—run seven days a week. I need to sit still.

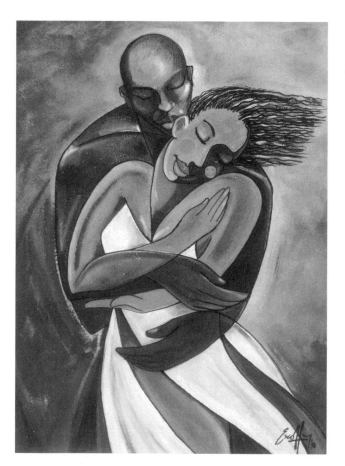

I think I've got another ten years left. Then I'll be ready for my second career. Maybe I'll go on to be a teacher or a therapist. Something where I can sit down. I think I want to sit down for the next twenty years.

The Embrace, *1996.*

MICHAEL ESCOFFERY

ART RESOURCE

DON'T CHANGE A HAIR FOR ME

In the 1920s, during the sculptor Augusta Savage's stay in Paris, she straightened her hair with the flame from a Sterno cup and the straightening comb she'd brought with her from the United States. One day, a black girl from the Caribbean island of Martinique observed Savage and asked the artist to help her straighten her own bushy hair. The girl was getting ready for a big date with her French boyfriend, who seemed on the verge of proposing. Savage was happy to oblige.

Later that evening, however, there was a frantic pounding at the sculptor's door. There, the Martinican girl stood sobbing on the threshhold. Her Frenchman, she told Savage, had been furious about the appearance of her straightened hair, and had refused to be seen with her on the street. Now, she lamented, she was ruined forever.

Savage soothed the girl and told her not to worry. With a quick dunk of the girl's head in water, her hair was back to its original, bushy state. The next day the girl was singing a happy tune again.

—Blanche Ferguson, *Countee Cullen and the Negro Renaissance*

When Worlds Collide

he borders of Africa and the Americas touch through transat-lantic journeys linked by lengths of hair. Cultures combine, con-verge, clash. Some traditions die, and the seeds of new ones are sown. The Afro blossomed on the New York black art scene in the late fifties and early sixties. Both a bohemian fashion statement and a symbol of solidarity with Africa's independence movements, the Afro style was being worn by black women on both sides of the Atlantic. In many ways, we continue to mirror one another.

FIRST 'FRO'S

"In the early '50s, throughout my elementary and junior high school years, my mother wore her hair natural and regularly wore African dress. There were perhaps eight other black women in the United States under 100 years old who wore their hair that way at that time. My mother knew them all."

—Guy Johnson, Maya Angelou's son.

5 MORE EARLY AFRO WEARERS

Margaret Burroughs
Odetta
Abbey Lincoln
Nina Simone
Cecily Tyson

THE CURSE (AND REDEMPTION) OF SHORT HAIR
Thomas "Taiwo" Duvall

Juanita Davis was a lively topic in 1942 when I was in grade school. She had practically no hair! It was basically a fuzz. The kids said her hair was so short

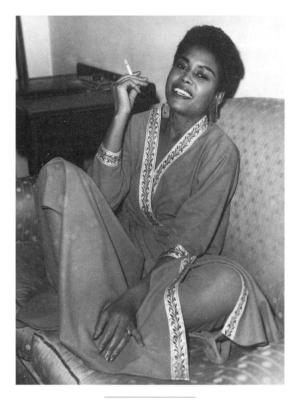

Abbey Lincoln in 1958.

HULTON-DEUTSCH COLLECTION/CORBIS

eceeeee

▪ 1960 ▪

LOST IN THE TRANSLATION

South African singer Miriam Makeba comes to the United States for the first time to perform. On the day of the opening, she is taken to Harlem to get her hair done for the show. The look of this time is straight and elegant, like that of the rising star Diahann Carroll. But Makeba likes her hair the way it is: short and wooly. Rose Morgan, Joe Lewis's former wife and the owner of the city's top black salon, straightens Makeba's hair. The young African singer thanks her but cannot bear to look at herself in the mirror. She is too afraid: "When I get back to the hotel and see what she has done to me, I cry and cry. This is not me. I put my head in the hot water and I wash it and wash it."

—*Makeba: My Story* by Miraim Makeba with James Hall

and nappy that every time her mother would buy her a new bow ribbon, she would have to send her to the store to buy glue to glue it on with! I felt so sorry for her, you could see she was not taking it well.

Juanita was a skinny girl, very plain looking, loped when she walked, never smiled, and had an aura of poverty. She was madly in love with John Smith (the handsome boy with the real curly hair), and he wouldn't give her the time of day. She was so mad at his aloofness that she decided to pick a fight with him and made the mistake of trying to take her coat off first. That's when he hit her. Her arms were caught in her coat and she was defenseless. She fell over backwards and her butt hit the ground. She was crushed. I felt bad for her; she was sitting on the ground soaked with tears. Nobody moved to help her. John Smith laughed out loud and walked away.

I helped Juanita to her feet, brushed her off, and helped her put her coat back on right. She never looked at me and she never said thanks. I told John Smith, "You didn't have to hit her! She was only trying to get your attention!" He looked at me like I was crazy.

In the late 1950s, when I was a member of African drummer Olatunji's troupe, I knew black women who purposefully wore their hair like Juanita's with great nerve, verve, and pride. These were the first African-American women, in modern times, to appear in public "au naturel"—people like my friends Pearl Primus and the late Esther Rolle, who was from a family of entertainers and always wore the "natural" look. Among the other first women to wear close, cropped natural hairstyles were Izme Andrews, singer Abbey Lincoln (with whom I had the pleasure of recording Max Roach's "Freedom Now Suite"), the Dancing Derby sisters, Mrs. Amy Olatunji, dancer-writer Maya Angelou, and dancer Helena Walker, to name a few. I had the pleasure of working and traveling with them for many years. I found their natural look refreshing; it made their skin sparkle—all-in-all a healthy, wholesome look. To me it was a mark of intelligence. If only Juanita Davis could have been there!

HAIR HYSTERIA

S. Pearl Sharp

"They're killing me! Ten o'clock and I don't have the first shot." Agitated, the young director ran his fingers through his hair as he paced the hall outside the dressing rooms.

He had his problems, I had mine. They had put a Mary Poppins-looking wig on my head and I was not happy.

Once again, Hair and Fear had collided. The scene was a studio in New York City where we were filming a TV spot for Crisco Oil. Not just any spot. This was to be the first "all-black" television commercial, a direct result of the Civil Rights Movement, which demanded, among other things, more visibility for black Americans in national ad campaigns.

While our presence in commercials was not new, we were moving from the era of invisible black actors whose Caucasian features were their selling point to the "sidekick" period where black persons couldn't pitch a product unless a white person was with them.

The scene we were shooting was a small party. Procter and Gamble, the parent company of Crisco, thought the party should be integrated. It was 1969 and integration was the mantra of the politically correct. But producer Percy Hall of Compton Advertising, then one of the few black advertising executives in all of North America, had convinced P&G that two black women throwing a party in their own apartment might, integration notwithstanding, invite just their own folks.

It would be Percy's crazy and unguarded sense of humor that got us through the day, but when we met on the set at 7:30 that morning, he was already sweating.

"The Client" arrived from their Midwestern headquarters with fear on their faces. A small group of buttoned-down white folks, their job was to make sure

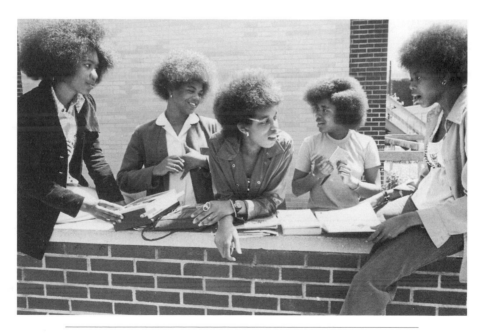

A moment in the early 1970s when everyone with hair to do so, wore a 'fro.

PHOTO: ROLAND FREEMAN

the commercial fit the P&G image and appealed to the widest range of consumers while offending no one.

So when Marcia McBroom, the other lead actress in the spot, and I made our first appearance in the wardrobe, hair, and makeup room for the shoot, there was an immediate huddle and flurry of whispers. Bad sign. We were sent back to the dressing room to wait.

About five minutes passed before the director appeared, "They, uh . . . It's uh. . . ." He was tall, white, a pleasant man with high energy. I could sense he was in a bind.

"It's the hair."

Marcia was wearing a "curly Afro," a 50/50 compromise between curl and kink. I was wearing a full "natural" Afro, picked and large.

"It's the hair," he repeated apologetically. "They're afraid the two Afros will appear too militant in the Southern market."

The "Southern market" has a notorious history relating to images of black women.

Singer Lena Horne, for example, the first African-American woman to have a long-term contract with a major Hollywood studio, was usually filmed in such a way that her scenes could be cut out if her presence offended Southern film censors. And diva Dorothy Dandridge starred in films that had two sets of advertising posters: one with her and one without her. So here on the brink of the "militant" '70s, when a clenched fist and the phrase "black power" were seen as threats, we knew exactly what was happening.

Over the next four hours things went from the unnecessary to the ridiculous, like putting me in that Mary Poppins wig. The Client was about to give it the stamp of approval until Percy saw me and laughed so hard they had to bring him some water.

So my 'fro was pinned back, then picked out again while Marcia was taxied home to get her straight-hair wig. One big 'fro, one black Suzy Wong, and the vote was split. Marcia went back to the curly 'fro while I donned the straight wig. Thumbs down. Then I was sent home to get my wig. It was sort of reddish-brown-curly-straight, crumpled in the back of a drawer, and wig curls get real territorial when not being used. I dropped it on them just as it was.

At half past noon we were back where we started. We were also half an hour from lunch and the director still didn't have his first shot, but he was getting his first ulcer. Percy had sweated off a couple of pounds, the crew was taking snide bets on when we'd get started, and the woman responsible for keeping the Crisco fried-chicken camera perfect was about to lose it. Thousands of dollars were going up in hair every minute. Under this mounting pressure, the group finally agreed that the South would neither fall nor rise again over this commercial, and Afros would be OK.

As we headed for the dressing rooms to do final prep, a blonde client, who had been most controlling and whiny all morning, piped up.

"Well, I don't know. If one of the girls could just pull the front of her hair down, to make some sort of bangs . . . Wouldn't bangs be lovely?"

That did it. Any requisite congeniality was gone and in a second they were all screaming at each other.

The director stomped into the dressing room, nostrils flared, eyes blazing, teeth clenched.

"It! Will! Take! You! At! Least! Two! Hours! Tofixyourhairagain!" His head bobbed up and down like a puppet as he directed our response.

"Oh, yes! Absolutely," Marcia and I moaned dramatically, raising our voices so they would float out to The Client. "Two hours, maybe three."

The director spun around, stomped out of the room like a World Series umpire on the third out, and shouted, "They've all got hair. Let's shoot this motherfucker!"

Within minutes the cameras were rolling. And quite simply, television history was made as two black women fried up some chicken and threw a party, in their own home, in their own hair.

REMEMBER THE TIME

Big bushy Afros on the sisters and hardbop in the air. . . . Hair was pride you could grow . . . when you pulled the sisters to your chest it was pride you could rest your face in. My wife, Karen, had a 'fro the size of a small umbrella. A strong, proud woman whose beauty I would forever endeavor to earn.

—A. B. Spelman

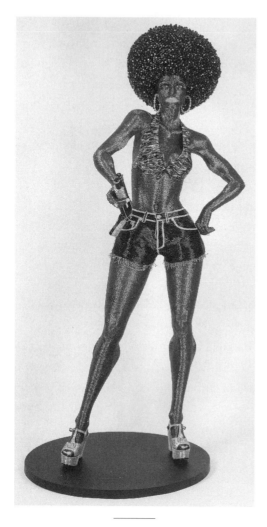

Supersister.
Bead sculpture inspired by Pam Grier.
LIZA LOU

By the early 1970s, on the eve of the Afro's ultimate demise, the whole "natural" movement took another turn. First, the Afro began to lose its specific political meaning, or at least the connection to black nationalist politics seemed to fade into the background

—Robin D. G. Kelley,
"Nap Time: Historicizing the Afro,"
Fashion Theory, Vol. 1

AFRO IMAGES: POLITICS, FASHION AND NOSTALGIA
Angela Y. Davis

Not long ago, I attended a collaborative performance in San Francisco by women presently or formerly incarcerated in the County Jail and Bay Area women performance artists. After the show, I went backstage to the "green room," where the women inmates, guarded by deputy sheriffs stationed outside the door, were celebrating with their families and friends. Having worked with some of the women at the jail, I wanted to congratulate them on the show. One woman introduced me to her brother, who at first responded to my name with a blank stare. The woman admonished him: "You don't know who Angela Davis is? You should be ashamed." Suddenly a flicker of recognition flashed across his face. "Oh," he said, "Angela Davis—the Afro."

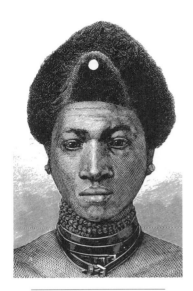

*The round Afro that we know
had angular antecedents.
(From* 400 Years Without a
Comb, *by Willie Morrow)*

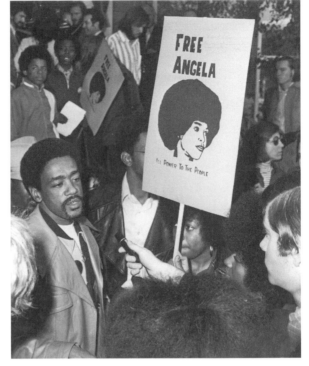

"Free Angela" Davis Rally.

AP WORLD WIDE PHOTOS

Such responses are commonplace rather than exceptional, and it is both humiliating and humbling to discover that a generation following the events which constructed me as a public personality, I am remembered as a hairdo. It is humiliating because it reduces a politics of liberation to a politics of fashion; it is humbling because such encounters with the younger generation demonstrate the fragility and mutability of historical images, particularly those associated with African-American history. This encounter with the young man who identified me as "the Afro" reminded me of a recent article in *The New York Times Magazine* which listed me as one of the fifty most influential fashion (read: hairstyle) trendsetters over the last century.[1] I continue to find it ironic that the popularity of the "Afro" is attributed to me, when, in actuality, I was emulating a whole host of women—both public figures and women I encountered in my daily life— when I began to wear my hair natural in the late sixties.

But it is not merely the reduction of historical politics to contemporary fashion that infuriates me. Especially disconcerting is the fact that the distinction of being known as "the Afro" is largely a result of a particular economy of journalistic images in which mine is one of the relatively few that has survived the last two decades. Or perhaps the very segregation of those photographic images caused mine to enter into the then-dominant journalistic culture precisely by virtue of my presumed "criminality." In any case, it has survived, disconnected from the historical context in which it arose, as fashion. Most young African-Americans who are familiar with my name and twenty-five-year-old image have encountered photographs and film/video clips largely in music videos, and in black history montages in popular books and magazines. In the interpretive context within which they learn to situate these photographs, the most salient element of the image is the hairstyle, understood less as a political statement than as fashion.

The unprecedented contemporary circulation of the photographic and filmic images of African-Americans has multiple and contradictory implications. On the one hand, it holds the promise of visual memory of older and departed generations—both well-known figures and people who may not have achieved public prominence. However, there is also the danger that this historical memory becomes ahistorical and apolitical. "Photographs are relics of the past," John Berger has written. They are

> *. . . traces of what has happened. If the living take that past upon themselves, if the past becomes an integral part of the process of people making their own history, then all photographs would acquire a living context, they would continue to exist in time, instead of being arrested moments.[2]*

In the past, I have been rather reluctant to reflect in more than a casual way about the power of the visual images by which I was represented during the period of my trial. Perhaps this is due to my unwillingness to confront those images as having to some extent structured my experiences during that era. The recent recycling of some of these images in contexts that privilege the "Afro" as fashion—revolutionary glamour—has led me to consider them both in the historical context in which they were first produced (and in which I first experienced them) and within the "historical" context in which they often are presented today as "arrested moments."

In September 1969, the University of California Regents fired me from my post in the Philosophy Department at UCLA because of my membership in the Communist Party. The following summer, charges of murder, kidnapping, and conspiracy were brought against me in connection with my activities on behalf of George Jackson and the Soledad Brothers. The circulation of various photographic images of me—taken by journalists, undercover policemen, and movement activists—played a major role in both the mobilization of public opinion against me *and* the development of a campaign that was ultimately responsible for my acquittal.

Twenty-five years later, many of these photographs are being recycled and recontextualized in ways that are at once exciting and disturbing. With the first public circulation of my photographs, I was intensely aware of the invasive and transformative power of the camera and of the ideological contextualization of my images that left me with little or no agency. On the one hand I was portrayed as a conspiratorial and monstrous Communist, i.e., anti-American, whose unruly natural hairdo symbolized black militancy, i.e., anti-whiteness. Some of the first hate mail I received tended to collapse "Russia" and "Africa." I was told to "go back to Russia" and often in the same sentence (in connection with a reference to my hair) to "go back to Africa." On the other hand, sympathetic portrayals tended to interpret the image—almost inevitably one with my mouth wide open—as that of a charismatic and raucous revolutionary ready to lead the masses into battle. Since I considered myself neither monstrous nor charismatic, I felt fundamentally betrayed on both accounts: violated on the first account, and deficient on the second.

When I was fired by the UC Regents in 1969, an assortment of photographs appeared in various newspapers, magazines and on television throughout that year. However, it was not until felony charges were brought against me in connection with the Marin County shootout that the photographs became what Susan Sontag has called a part of "the general furniture of the environment."[3] As such, they truly began to frighten me. A cycle of terror was initiated by the decision of the F.B.I. to declare me one of the country's ten most wanted criminals. Although I had been underground for more than a month before I actually saw the photographs the F.B.I. had decided to use on the poster, I had to picture how they might portray me as I attempted to create for myself an appearance that would be markedly different from the one defined as armed and dangerous. The props I used consisted of a wig with straight hair, long false lashes, and more eyeshadow, liner, and blush than I had ever before imagined wearing in public. Never having seriously attempted to present myself as glamorous, it seemed to me that the glamour was the only look that might annul the likelihood of being perceived as a revolutionary. It never could have occurred to me that the same "revolutionary" image I then sought to camouflage with glamour would be turned, a generation later, into glamour and nostalgia.

After the F.B.I. poster was put on display in post offices, other government buildings, and on the television program *The F.B.I.*, *Life* magazine came out with a provocative issue featuring a cover story on me. Illustrated with photographs from my childhood years through the UCLA firing, the article probed the reasons for my supposedly abandoning a sure trajectory toward fulfillment of the middle-class American dream in order to lead the unpredictable life of a "black revolutionary." Considering the vast circulation of this pictorial magazine,[4] I experienced something akin to what Barthes was referring to when he wrote:

> *I feel that the Photograph creates my body or mortifies it, according to its caprice (apology of this mortiferous power: certain Communards paid with their lives for their willingness or even their eagerness to pose on the barricades: defeated, they were recognized by Thiers's police and shot, almost every one).*[5]

The life-sized head shot on the cover of the magazine would be seen by as many people, if not more, than the much smaller portraits on the F.B.I. poster. Having confronted my own image in the news store where I purchased the magazine, I was convinced that the F.B.I chief J. Edgar Hoover had conspired in the appearance of that cover story. More than anything else, it seemed to me to be a magnification and elaboration of the wanted poster. Moreover, the text of the story gave a rather convincing explanation as to why the pictures should be associated with arms and danger.

The photograph on the cover of my autobiography,[6] published in 1974, was taken by the renowned photographer Phillipe Halsman. When Toni Morrison—who was my editor—and I entered his studio, the first question he asked us was whether we had brought the black leather jacket. He assumed, it turned out, that he was to re-create with his camera a symbolic visual representation of black militancy: leather jacket (uniform of the Black Panther Party), Afro hairdo, and raised fist. We had to persuade him to photograph me in a less predictable posture. As recently as 1993, the persisting persuasiveness of those visual stereotypes was made clear to me when I had to insist that Anna Deavere Smith rethink her representation of me in *Fires in the Mirror,* which initially relied upon a black leather jacket as her main prop.

So far, I have concentrated primarily on my own responses to those photographic images, which may not be the most interesting or productive way to approach them. While the most obvious evidence of their power was the part they played in structuring people's opinions about me as a "fugitive" and a political prisoner, their more subtle and wide-ranging effect was the way they served as generic images of black women who wore their hair "natural." From the constant stream of stories I have heard during the last twenty-four years (and continue to hear), I infer that definitely hundreds—perhaps even thousands—of Afro-wearing black women were accosted, harassed, and arrested by police, F.B.I., and immigration agents during the two months I spent underground. One woman, who told me that she hoped she could serve as a "decoy" because of her light skin and big natural, was obviously conscious of the way the photographs—circulating within a highly charged racialized context—constructed generic representations of young black women. Consequently, the photographs identified vast numbers of my black female contemporaries who wore natural (whether light- or dark-skinned) as targets of repression. This is the hidden historical context that lurks behind the continued association of my name with the Afro.

A young former student of mine has been wearing an Afro during the last few months. Rarely a day passes, she has told me, when she is not greeted with cries of "Angela Davis" from total strangers. Moreover, during the months preceding the writing of this article, I have received an astounding number of requests for interviews from journalists doing stories on "the resurgence of the Afro." A number of the requests were occasioned by a layout in the fashion section of the March 1994 issue of *Vibe* magazine titled "Free Angela: Actress Cynda Williams as Angela Davis, a fashion revolutionary." The spread consists of eight full-page photos of Cynda Williams (known for her role as the singer in Spike Lee's *Mo Better Blues)* in poses that parody photographs taken of me during the early 1970s. The work of stylist Patty Wilson, the layout is described as "'docufashion' because it uses modern clothing to mimic Angela Davis's look from the '70s."[7]

Some of the pictures are rather straightforward attempts to re-create press photos taken at my arrest, during the trial, and after my release. Others can be characterized as pastiche,[8] drawing elements, such as leather-jacketed black men, from contemporary stereotypes of the sixties to seventies era of black militancy. These include an arrest scene, with the model situated between two uniformed policemen and wearing an advertised black satin blouse (reminiscent of the top I was wearing on the date of my arrest). Like her hair, the advertised glasses are amazingly similar to the ones I wore. There are two courtroom scenes in which Williams wears an enormous Afro wig and advertised see-through minidresses and, in one of them, handcuffs. Yet another revolves around a cigar-smoking, bearded man dressed in fatigues with a gun holster around his waist, obviously meant to evoke Che Guevara. (Even the fatigues can be purchased from Cheap Jack's!) There is no such thing as subtlety in these photos. Because the point of this fashion spread is to represent the clothing associated with revolutionary movements of the early seventies as revolutionary fashion in the nineties, the six-tieth anniversary logo of the Communist Party has been altered in one of the photos to read 1919-1971 (instead of 1979). And the advertised dress in the photo for which this logo is a backdrop is adorned with pin-on buttons reading "Free All Political Prisoners."

The photographs I find most unsettling, however, are the two small head-shots of Williams wearing a huge Afro wig on a reproduction of the F.B.I. wanted poster that is otherwise unaltered except for the words "FREE AN-GELA" in bold red print across the bottom of the document. Despite the fact that the inordinately small photos do not really permit much of a view of the clothing Williams wears, the tops and glasses (again quite similar to the ones I wore in the two imitated photographs) are listed as purchasable items. This is the most blatant example of the way the particular history of my legal case is emp-tied of all content so that it can serve as a commodified backdrop for advertising. The way in which this document provided a historical pretext for something akin to a reign of terror for countless young black women is effectively erased by its use as a prop for selling clothes and promoting a seventies fashion nostalgia. What is also lost in this nostalgic surrogate for historical memory—in these "ar-rested moments," to use John Berger's words—is the activist involvement of vast numbers of black women in movements that are now represented with even greater masculinist contours than they actually exhibited at the time.

Without engaging the numerous debates occasioned by Frederic Jameson's paper "Postmodernsim and Consumer Society,"[9] I would like to suggest that this analysis of "nostalgia films" and their literary counterparts that are "historical novels in appearance only," might provide a useful point of departure for an interpretation of this advertising genre call "docufashion," as yet a further site for the proliferation of nostalgic images. "[W]e seem condemned to seek the historical past," Jameson writes, "through our own pop images and stereotypes about that past, which itself remains forever out of reach."[10] Perhaps by also taking up John Berger's call for an "alternative photography" we might develop strategies for engaging with photographic images like the ones I have evoked, by actively seeking to transform their interpretive contexts in education, popular culture, the media, community organizing, and so on. Particularly in relation to African-American historical images, we need to find ways of incorporating them into "social and political memory, instead of using [them] as a substitute which encourages the atrophy of such memory."[11]

Notes

[1] "50 Who Mattered Most," *New York Times Magazine*, October 24, 1993, pp. 122-25.

[2] John Berger, *About Looking*, New York: Pantheon Books, 1980, p. 57.

[3] Susan Sontag, *On Photography*, New York: Farrar, Straus and Giroux, 1978, p. 27.

[4] During the 1960s, *Life* magazine had a circulation of approximately 40 million. (Gisele Freund, *Photography and Society*, Boston: David R. Goddine, 1980, p. 143)

[5] Roland Barthes, *Camera Lucida*, New York: Hill and Lang, 1981, p. 11.

[6] *Angela Y. Davis: An Autobiography*, New York: Random House, 1974.

[7] *Vibe*, Volume 2, No. 2, March 1994, p. 16.

[8] I use the term "pastiche" both in the usual sense of a potpourri of disparate ingredients and in the sense in which Frederic Jameson uses it. "Pastiche is, like parody, the imitation of a peculiar or unique style, the wearing of a stylistic mask, speech in a dead language but it is a neutral practice of such mimicry, without parody's ulterior motive, without the satirical impulse, without laughter. . . . Pastiche is a black parody, parody that has lost its sense of humor . . ." Frederic Jameson, "Postmodernism and Consumer Society" in Hal

Foster, ed., *The Anti-Aesthetic: Essays of Postmodern Culture*. Port Townsend, Washington: Bay Press, 1983, p 114.

[9] Jameson's essay has appeared in several versions. The one I have consulted is referenced in note 8. I thank Victoria Smith for suggesting that I reread this essay in connection with the *Vibe* story.

[10] Jameson, p. 118.

[11] Berger, p. 58.

DAUGHTERS OF AFRICA
Evangeline Wheeler

I dressed in a bright colorful *boubou* featuring the president's wrinkled face against a blue-printed background and waited eagerly for my friends to pick me up. A cool breeze stirred in the doorway, so I extended my arms skyward, inviting it to caress my sticky underarms. I felt grateful that evening was falling after such a scorching day.

In a few minutes' time, my African friends and I would be off to Christmas Eve services at the Catholic Mission in Kagabandoro, a town in the Central African Republic. I'm not Catholic, but this celebration at the mission was the hottest ticket in town. After several months of living in my new village, I could speak Sango and bake corn bread on a kerosene stove. Before the ink had dried on my doctoral degree, I'd joined the Peace Corps and moved to a small town in the heart of the Motherland.

Like most of the rural women there with whom I lived and worked, I wore my hair in tiny, tight cornrows. The everyday style I preferred was simple, with the rows beginning at the baby hair on my forehead and trailing straight back to the kitchen. Usually I could count fourteen or fifteen of them. Many hot afternoons passed with my behind on the ground and my head wedged between the sturdy thighs of Solange, a teenager, as she skillfully braided my hair into a style that kept for weeks. Hair-braiding sessions took up many of those long afternoon hours after the cassava fields were tended and the midday meal eaten.

The city women who considered themselves more sophisticated than their village sisters clamored for the hair straighteners and extensions ("connections," the Kenyan women called them) that had become readily available, if expensive.

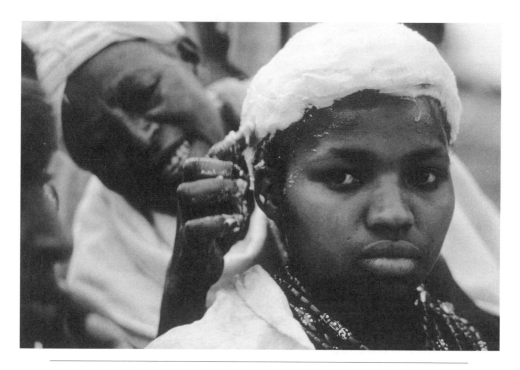

A young woman participating in a Dorze coming-of-age ceremony has butter, a rare and precious commodity for the group, applied to her hair to celebrate her femininity and sexuality.

JIM SUGAR PHOTOGRAPHY/CORBIS

Fashion magazines from Paris and the United States had influenced them. But I felt they were ignoring a cultural gift because the young women in the country-side were so skilled at creating the tiniest plaits in the most intricate patterns. This dimension of sharing in the care of the black female self served to bring us closer, and surviving the import of the perms and extensions, it remains a feature of the everyday life of many African women.

When my friends arrived, we walked the quarter mile to the church. Towns-people overflowed the grounds. They, like our little group, came chattering and preening, gossiping and laughing. Everyone was dressed in the best outfit she owned. Beautiful little girls sparkled in brightly colored dresses. Their intricate, complicated hairstyles affected me like artwork. The styles got more intriguing as my head pivoted from one child to the next—breathtaking braided patterns that demanded examination. Very unexpectedly, I began to cry, so moved was I by the physical beauty of dozens of lithe, confident African girls, all decked out in their prettiest dresses radiant with color, heads held proudly high, displaying the talent of the town's best braiders.

ON SHORT NAPPY HAIR AND THE BUSINESS OF BLACKNESS: FROM OHIO TO SOUTH AFRICA
Paitra D. Russell

I don't know what happened to NeNe's hair. One day she was wearing it pulled back, the next it had broken off down to the new growth. She got on the bus that day just like every other morning, but when she pulled her hood down, we all saw that her hair was perhaps half an inch long all over—and nappy— except for a long straight piece in the front that had remained intact.

My best friend Stephanie and I stared at the back of her head that morning and for a long time afterward, trying to figure out what had happened. An accident? Whacked off in a fight? Or just overprocessed back and forth—from a curl to a perm to a curl—to the point that it had given up and fallen out? Whatever the case, we knew this was not a look she had chosen voluntarily.

We were in high school, a time when looking "good" defined our very lives. Having short nappy hair essentially ruined a girl's chances of looking "good," and therefore of having a satisfying social life. My older and wiser friend Kim routinely summed up the importance of looking "good," and the requirements for it, in her descriptions of her boyfriends.

"He looks good, girl: he's light-skinned, got a curl, and pretty eyes, too."

"Pretty eyes" were those of any color other than the typical dark brown we all had. Kim herself had "pretty eyes." In her case, they were light brown. Really pretty eyes were green or hazel, even occasionally blue, but that was rare. "Pretty eyes" preferably went with light skin and "good hair," that is straight, wavy, or curly—anything but nappy—and impervious to the kinkifying effects of water and sweat. This allowed one to enjoy swim classes and house parties alike.

For those of us who did not have "good hair," however, a curl (Care-Free, California, or Quadra) was close enough. In the 1980s glamour was in, and everyone knew what it looked like. Angela Davis knew in 1970. Writing nearly a quarter century after going underground, she recalls choosing a disguise of glam-

THE BOONDOCKS

by AARON McGRUDER

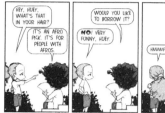
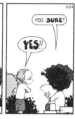
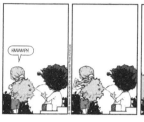
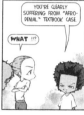

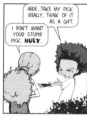
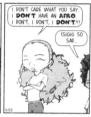
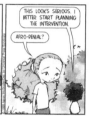

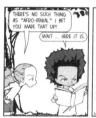
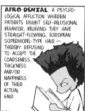
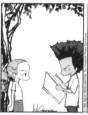
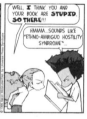

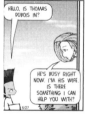
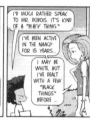
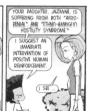
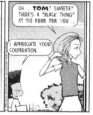

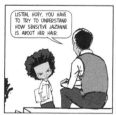
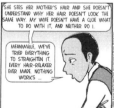
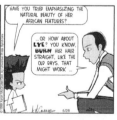

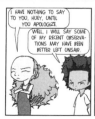
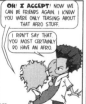
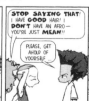
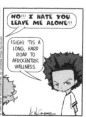

our because it was diametrically opposed to her well-publicized Afro. To simulate this glamour, Davis donned a wig of long, straight hair, false eyelashes, and heavy makeup. This, she wrote, "seemed to me . . . the only look that might annul the likelihood of being perceived as revolutionary."

In the fifteen years since Davis had fled the authorities, Black Power had gone underground and out of style, right along with Davis and her Afro. We eighties children longed for its antithesis—the sleek, wet look of shiny cars and drippy hair, as exemplified by Crockett and Tubbs every week on *Miami Vice,* our favorite television show. As Philip Michael Thomas (and his soul-singer looka-likes) came to embody ideal black manhood, weaves and colored contacts arrived to scoot black women along in our beauty quest. Early on, however, these fabu-lous products seemed available only to successful sisters in Los Angeles or Miami or some other place where the streets were lined with palm trees. Dark Ohio girls like me in dying industrial towns settled for a curl and TV.

One day NeNe and a boy called Dink got into it on the bus. I don't remem-ber what sparked their argument, but NeNe was winning. We all laughed as they hurled insults at each other. Then, sensing imminent defeat, Dink pulled out the heavy artillery: he called NeNe a bald bitch. It was an insult so vile that it si-lenced everybody except NeNe.

"I know I'm bald," she said. "You think I don't see myself in the mirror every morning?"

Well, what else could she say? Simply to maintain some dignity in the face of such an attack was no small feat. But she didn't have a retort, and none of us could help her. Not even a "Yo Mama" from an anonymous ally in the crowd could have eased the tension and made it all a game again. Dink had raised the stakes to something far beyond school-bus dozens. To respond in kind, NeNe would have had to call the size of Dink's penis into question—to assault his manhood in the same way that he had just erased her femininity. I would like to think that NeNe refused to stoop to his level and chose instead to dismiss the gravity of his comment through the simple act of agreement. To say "Yes. And?" as if he'd said nothing of importance at all. I suspect, however, that like the rest of us, NeNe was just too stunned to say anything else.

Calling NeNe a bitch was the least of it, even though "bitch" had not yet be-come (along with "ho") the standard reference to a black woman in the popular imagination of the gutter. While NeNe could have hit Dink for calling her a bitch, there was no defense against being bald. Dink might as well have been making fun of an amputee's missing limb, for short, nappy hair, like an amputation, was a tragedy. The long bang NeNe had continued to wear, the last remnant of a full head of sometimes-curly/sometimes-straight hair, operated like a ghost limb, reminding her, and everyone who stared, that once upon a time she had been normal.

As we got off the bus that morning, my friend Stephanie flicked one long fingernail hard against Dink's own bald head as a kind of reprimand. It was the best we could do.

Within a couple of years, curls went out, and like every other black girl I knew, I started wearing my hair straight again (albeit shaved in the back, asymmetrical on the sides, and crimped on top). "Bone Straight" (the name of a perm) became a compliment. The weaves and colored contacts so far out of reach in high school suddenly seemed to become generally available. And for those of us who couldn't approximate the hair-down-your-back look popularized in black music videos, there was the "wrap" to ensure that our hair would actually hang, perhaps even blow in the wind, if the ends cleared your chin.

I didn't think much about it at the time; then suddenly it was the nineties and black consciousness was back. Not the protest kind with marching and singing and some kind of legislative gesture toward social change. No, the new black consciousness was the consumption kind. It had us buying cowrie shells, imitation kente cloth and "It's a Black Thing" T-shirts. Weaves were forced to acquire texture, and everyone got braids. Who said long, store-bought hair bespoke a white mentality? Now one could have hair down one's back and be Afrocentric at the same time!

By 1994 naturals were everywhere in New York City, the cosmopolitan promised land to which I fled after eighteen mind-numbing years in Ohio. As I thought about it, I had never seen a woman with a natural who didn't look beautiful, self-confident, and powerful. I wanted that, too. I also wanted to prove to myself that I could completely kick the chemical habit, because I truly was addicted to having what comes with long, straight hair: the privilege to just be.

Are you with me?

Having long straight hair means your hair isn't an issue. It's just hair, like any(white)body's. Pull it back in a ponytail and go on about your business, your schoolwork, your career, your life. No one will even notice, or if they do, it's with admiration. If you are in an argument, no one will call you a long-haired bitch. So what black American woman in her right mind cuts off hair that reaches the bottom of her chin even after it's been curled? My hair was finally one length (long) and one texture (straight). I liked it. My friends liked it. My family liked it. My man liked it. But I'll tell you a secret: I wasn't happy. And if you've ever had long, relaxed hair, I suspect you already know why. First of all, the following sentences were part of my regular vocabulary:

I can't, I'm doing my hair that day.

and

I can't, I'm going to the hairdresser that day.

and

It's BURNING!

Also: money and time. The beauty salon is a place where one could easily spend 10 percent of one's time and 20 percent of one's money. Time is squandered flipping through old magazines, listening to AM radio, watching TV with no sound. I'd leave the shop with a shiny film on my face and a headache from the chemical burns, exacerbated by the blow dryer and curling iron, compounded by the smell of burned hair and aerosol sprays I'd been inhaling during my extended visit. In the summer the humidity outside was always higher than 5 percent, so by the time I got home it was the clock, my wallet, and two new pimples that indicated how I had spent the day. I tell you, I was living the Hegelian master/slave dialectic: I was no longer the master of my hair, I was a slave to it.

So on an early spring evening in 1994, I threw my lot in with the likes of NeNe and the millions of women walking around with short, nappy hair, either on purpose or as the result of some disastrous chemical overload. I took out the shoulder-length braids I'd been wearing for three months while my relaxer grew out, and went to a barbershop in Harlem. I told the barber, the only woman barber I'd ever seen, to cut my hair into a nice, round, graceful natural, leaving it a little higher on top. I laughed at the guys in the shop who warned—no begged—me not to do it: "Aw, girl, please don't cut all your hair off." "It's just hair," I told them, smiling. It would grow back if I let it.

I stared at Leslie, the friend I had brought along for moral support. She already had a natural, and it looked damned good. I looked to the expression on her face to reveal whether my head was misshapen or couldn't "carry" a natural because my face was too full, thin, round, square, wide, or narrow. In short, she would tell me if any of the excuses I and everyone else I knew used to explain why we couldn't "go natural" were valid. Leslie smiled encouragingly throughout the process. Zakia, the barber, worked intently and silently.

An hour later, I looked in the mirror and still liked myself. In fact, I was thrilled. I felt sophisticated and reborn, just like after getting any new style, but better, because somehow I had learned something important about myself: I was okay without chemicals. I didn't need straight hair to be happy and smart and self-confident. On our way over to Sylvia's, the famous soul food restaurant, to celebrate, I marveled at how sensual the cool air felt against my newly exposed scalp. Sexy!

Before I got my hair cut, I hadn't paid much attention to the Nation of Israel. I'd seen them preaching at the Fulton Street Mall in Brooklyn, or on 125th Street in Harlem. Their style of dress seemed vaguely medieval: loose pants tucked into high black boots, tunic shirts, and thick leather belts with a huge silver Star of David on the buckle. Once as I passed by, they tossed a painting of a blond, blue-eyed Jesus to the ground, shouting, "Jesus was a faggot!" But beyond this I took no notice of them. It was New York, after all.

But after the haircut I had several run-ins with the Nation of Israel. My hairstyle agitated them, and invariably one of them would make some disparaging remark: Why are you trying to look like a man? Why don't you put on a dress? And once when Leslie and I walked past them together on our way to a movie, they taunted, "Lesbians are going to hell! Even the black ones!"

I should have laughed, but I was outraged that a man wearing pantaloons and a ponytail would dare make assumptions about my sexual orientation because of my appearance. I challenged him on pan-Africanist grounds, an argument I assumed he would understand: We were getting back to our roots.

"Haven't you ever been to Africa?" I said.

"We aren't African," he replied. "We are Asiatic."

Oh.

We listened in confusion as he shouted Bible verses at us to "prove" that women should be submissive to men. We figured he had singled us out because two black women walking down the street together—while wearing short naturals—constituted some sort of violation (in much the same way that "driving while black" has become reason enough to be stopped by traffic cops). He and his friends were determined to show us the error of our ways. "Let the women learn in silence!" one shouted at us, gesturing toward the women who sat at their feet in long white shifts, heads bowed and covered. "God doesn't talk to women," another said.

But they'd picked the wrong sister to argue scripture with. Leslie had been memorizing scripture since she was a child. She was in seminary, and knew the Bible like the back of her hand. She reminded this man that as an Israelite he should be using a Hebrew Bible, and if he knew Hebrew, he'd know that the Hebrew word for God was not masculine and therefore should not have been translated into English as "He." It wasn't even singular. But when you get intellectual with a fascist, sexist, homophobic lunatic—well, all that's left is to become violent. So the man balled up his fists and screamed, "When God comes back, women are going to be beaten into their places for all eternity!!"

That was our cue to leave.

Fortunately, this experience was not the typical response to my hair. More often than not I'd get a nod and a smile, from women and men. Brothers with locks started noticing me. My white colleagues thought it was "cool." But . . . whether it was viewed as positive or negative, the fact was that my hair had become an issue. That confrontation on the corner of Fifty-sixth and Broadway, which left me trembling and weak with anger and incredulity and yes, fear, reminded me why I'd needed moral support in the barbershop to begin with. I wasn't just exercising my right to choose one of a million styles available to black women. I was thrusting myself into a position to see a whole world of ideas about how to act, dress, and look—rules I'd always followed even though I didn't think they were there. And the view from that position is frightening.

Friends and relatives kept asking, Why? They had to know what statement I was making. Was I coming out of the closet? Rebelling against authority? Rejecting a white standard of beauty? No one had asked why I dumped Jheri Curl goop on my head, to the detriment of an untold number of shirts, jackets, and pillowcases. No one asked why I grew my hair long and straightened it with chemicals, which deconstruct and reconstitute it at the molecular level. No one asked why I paid $250 and sat for eleven hours while two women weaved five pounds of synthetic material into my hair and then burned off the ends with a lighter.

But purposely wearing short, nappy hair? Now that was cause for concern. Even in the midst of abundant kente, cowrie, mudcloth, and knowing the ancient Egyptian word for "hello," short nappy hair is another issue entirely. I was so intrigued by this phenomenon that I wrote my master's thesis on it. And the deeper I got into the subject, the more complicated and frightening the whole business became. Because make no mistake: Hair is, indeed, a business, one that I investigated during fieldwork in South Africa for my doctoral dissertation.

A few months before those men in the Nation of Israel suggested I get back into my rightful place beneath their knee-high boots, non-white South Africans celebrated getting out from under the boot of the Afrikaner Nationalist Party government. Shortly afterward, black-owned corporations began announcing plans to expand into the newly freed, predominantly black South African market. With the political struggle over, in theory, African Americans could build mutually beneficial economic partnerships with our newly liberated brothers and sisters.

Three years after that nation's first free political elections, I found myself in the "new" South Africa, hoping to determine why new hair salons offering creme relaxers from the United States were popping up faster than new houses with running water. About the only thing as popular as Dark-N-Lovely was hydroquinone, the infamous skin lightener. I learned this after discussing my research with several women who immediately informed me that hair was not an issue at all—it was skin I should be looking at. So I did, and discovered that both skin lightening and hair straightening are parallel practices of "aesthetic assimilation," and are exploited by South African vendors and American corporations alike.

Skin-bleaching creams are so popular that the press regularly runs features on women who have permanently disfigured themselves by improperly using them. Skin lighteners were banned in South Africa in the 1980s because of the liver damage hydroquinone can cause. Since then, however, that product has flourished on the "black market" (a most unfortunate pun). Street vendors and sympathetic nurses provide the public with the goods. So two-thirds of the holy trinity of straight hair, light skin, and light eyes is readily available for a small fee. Colored contacts can't be far behind.

A popular black South African magazine, *Drum,* ran a couple of articles on the dangers of skin lightening while I was there. One, called "Safe Way to a Lighter Complexion," managed to reinforce the message that light skin is desirable even while discouraging women from using creams. In the center spread, a woman holds a plain tube of some substance under the heading: "A cream for a lighter skin. . . . Experts tell how to lighten and protect your face from the sun." Though the article suggests that skin-lightening creams are bad, it supports the notion that light skin itself is good, with statements like "some people still see themselves as 'too black' and try [skin-lightening creams and] other dangerous methods. But a safe sunblock does the job." The implicit message, of course, is that there is a job that needs to be done.

The article also points to some of the perceived purveyors of a particular look. One doctor blames the media for Africans' desire for lighter skin: "Although they push the 'black is beautiful' slogan, the models and pin-ups they choose are often women with light skin and a Western appearance," he says. Don't be misled: "Western" doesn't necessarily mean "white." It is often synonymous with "American," and according to the South Africans I've talked to, African Americans are much more American than African. From our music and speech to the way we walk and dance, we embody "the West." The article in *Drum* declares (rather disdainfully) that "African-Americans can get anything they want: from artificial skin colors to replacements for hair, face, nose, hips and lips" through a $44 million medical and cosmetics industry.

Before I went to South Africa, I thought that I would be able to blend into the black South African scenery as long as I hid my American accent. But before I even opened my mouth, South Africans knew that I wasn't from there. When I asked one friend about this, he said the first time he looked at me, he immediately thought, "That's not black." He identified my walk, bone structure, and hairstyle as the primary giveaways. My "Afrocentric" twists, which had evolved from my 1994 natural, were decidedly "Western" in South Africa. As disconcerting as it may be, the truth of the matter is that what we think is a "black thing" in the States is often an "American thing" when viewed from the continent.

Like most of the world, South Africa imports much of its entertainment from the United States. A virtual African-American world is represented through American media. That imaged presence is a highly stylized one, and the means to attain the "look" are also being profitably imported.

In a *Black Enterprise* magazine article detailing the international expansion of African-American-owned corporations, an executive at Pro-Line, a corporation which produces a popular hair relaxer, says the company targets countries "where blacks tend to assimilate to the dominant [white] culture." England is described as the "best" market because there is a "high literacy rate, a high enough income and an aesthetic consciousness about what is going on both [in the United States] and in Britain." Though the company's executives admit the need for "sensitivity" to the preferences of people in international markets where stylistic demands are different, the ultimate goal is to profitably "export our [African-American] culture."

We seem to be doing a fairly good job of it. South Africa's black hair and cosmetics industry grew from about 250 million rand (rough exchange rate) per year in 1990 to nearly a billion rand per year by 1998. When Procter and Gamble decided to get into the black hair-care market in 1997, it chose South Africa, not the United States, as the entry point. In Gaborone, capitol of the neighboring country, Botswana, high school girls are quitting school en masse to become cosmetologists, hoping to get rich. While braiding is still at least as popular as relaxing, I have a feeling that if the corporate missionaries preaching the gospel of glamour have their way, that won't be for long. Maybe relaxers are a natural coefficient to democracy, and "aesthetic consciousness" the postrevolutionary equivalent to political activism. Under apartheid, I suppose, no one had a choice but to have nappy hair, but now, all those previously neglected heads can be as chic in their freedom as those across the Atlantic, or as the models in *Ebony South Africa*. It is apparently much easier to create the "look" of sophistication and progress than the material trappings of it.

The "look" is completed by the sound. I was never more surprised to find (black) "America" in South Africa, as when, while listening to Good Hope FM (a radio station where DJs have American accents and names like "Kick Ass Kenny"), I heard a caller sending "shout outs" to his "homies."

"They're all West Coast homies," he added.

I was awestruck, as much by the African-American slang as by the reference to an East Coast/West Coast hip-hop rivalry that makes no sense in South Africa. "America" is indeed everywhere in South Africa, particularly in the realm of popular culture, and it often has specifically black referents: a plethora of African-American sitcoms and music videos on television, hip-hop and old-

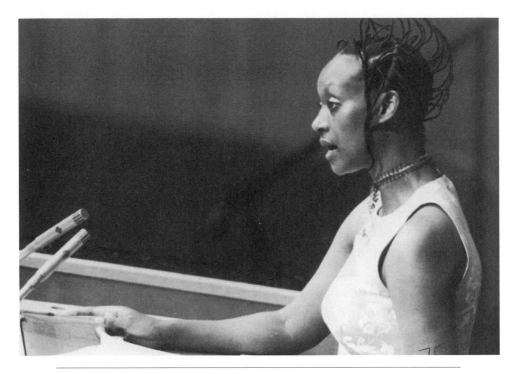

Elizabeth Bagaaya, a foreign minister from Uganda, addresses the United Nations.

BETTMAN/CORBIS

school soul on local radio stations, oversize jeans and backward baseball caps on teenage bodies.

There was a time when I would have found all this diasporic, transatlantic cultural mixing a testament to black creativity. Now I fear it is nothing more than the end product of market-hungry capitalism, eagerly proffering superficial representations of what it means to be black in America for the sake of profit in America *and* Africa.

Not long after I got to South Africa, I heard a joke from another African-American student. He got it from his brother in New York City, who apparently was unaware of the proliferation of hair-straightening practices throughout southern Africa and across the continent: "Africa: where all the women wear flat-tops."

How appropriate. America regularly portrays Africa as a region defined and characterized entirely by the tragedies of famine, war, disease, and poverty. It is not surprising that we would portray African women as suffering from the tragedy of short nappy hair as well. So, it seems that Dink's insult is alive and well.

HAIR GOES TO COLLEGE

As reported in a *Wall Street Journal* article about the "Black Hair as Culture and History" course at Stanford University, Professor Kennell Jackson asks if anyone has experienced "A Black Hair Event" recently. One student pipes up from the back of the room, noting that Juliette Lewis, a white actress, attended the Academy Awards ceremony with her hair cornrowed. "That's a good one," Professor Jackson agrees. "Any others?"

DECKED OUT

Slave ship captain J. G. Stedman wrote in his *Narrative of a Five Years' Expedition against the Revolted Negroes of Surinam* that no sooner had a ship arrived than all the Africans were led on deck, where they shaved each other's hair "in different figures of stars, half-moons," and such. With no razors at their disposal, they did this "by the help of a broken bottle and without soap."

SMOOTH HEATED STONES AND SUNLIGHT SOAP
Rosalie Kiah

On this August 1996 day in the Southern Hemisphere, there was a noticeable chill in the air. Winter was lasting a little longer than usual. The students strolling to classes wore baggy pants, sweat shirts, and Reeboks. With its modern buildings and spacious well-kept grounds, it could have been a university anywhere, but this was the first day of classes at the University of Botswana in southern Africa and the beginning of my two year stay as a Fulbright Scholar. I was here to teach literature of the African diaspora and a first-year course in communications skills.

As I walked to class that first day, I noticed the female students, and I was particularly struck by their hairstyles. They were as varied as the spectrum of skin colors. Some styles I recognized from the United States, like the tiny tight braids worn so elegantly by *Essence* editor Susan Taylor. I also saw the familiar style of hair swept up in a sleek cornrow that forms a basket at the crown of the head. Perhaps, like African-American women, these young women harbored obsessions about flowing, cascading hair, because there was plenty of l-o-n-g hair on their heads. I had to restrain myself because I wanted to ask questions straight away about some of the more unusual styles, but I knew that there would be plenty of time for this.

As the semester progressed, so did rapport, and the students and I talked freely about our respective cultures. I brought with me fifty or more back and current issues of *Ebony* and *Essence* magazines, which I made available in my office for students. They loved these publications, and my shelves were always bare. Certain issues were more popular than others, and it was apparent from the condition of returned issues that they had gone through many hands. The magazines that seemed to be most popular were the ones with Halle Berry on the covers.

One of the things I noticed most was how the hairstyles of some students changed from day to day, unlike at home. In the States, when black women made the move to extensions or a wig, that would be the style they wore for a while. Not so with these young sisters. So when it came to trying to learn students' names by making associations with their hairstyles, I found myself at a disadvantage. For example, Busi Manana, a very attractive student from Swaziland, and Katanego Nkoko from Botswana might have flowing extensions when class met on Monday, but when the class met again on Wednesday, these ladies would have relaxed their hair and be sporting a different 'do. And so it went.

One day some young women would come to class dressed to the nines, with their hair incongruously done in the juvenile three-plait style that I much despised as a child (one big plait hanging down the front left side, hair parted down the back with a plait on either side). Or they would have so much added hair that it was difficult for them to keep it out of their eyes as they wrote or read.

Because of the close proximity of Johannesburg ("the L.A. of Africa") to

Botswana, the university students read the South African edition of *Ebony* and watched BET-type shows, where fabulously talented young women in designer jeans and beaded skirts and expensive imported platform shoes strutted their stuff. Their heads were shaved, braided, or Afro-natural. When I asked several of the students where they got their ideas for hairstyles, the majority said the media.

Above all, that the style of choice was the simple cornrow, a style most indigenous to Africa. The students sometimes augmented them with long and short extensions, and braid bits littered walkways and grounds throughout the campus. One afternoon I counted at least a dozen of these little extension pieces on the ground as I walked home from classes.

It was not uncommon to see hair being braided between classes as the "client" sat on a campus bench reading her textbook and the "operator" plied her craft. Students said they preferred braided styles over others because braids make the hair grow thick and long.

I noticed that during the fall and winter (May through August), most women wore the heavy, thick braids that resembled twisted rope. Some of my students and colleagues in the English Department told me that these braids provide a source of heat as well as protection from the dust of the semi-desert climate.

I received quite a few comments from my students and colleagues about my own hair, which was relaxed. Tawana, my hairdresser in Norfolk, Virginia, had given me a touch-up before I left for Botswana, but there was nothing really special about my hair. I did not have a knockout cut, just plain relaxed hair. But Bono, the technician in the Educational Technology Center on campus, always complimented me on my hair. This made me feel really good because I had quite a few "bad-hair days" after the relaxer needed to be touched up. Bono would say the same thing every time I saw her: "Dumela Mma Kiah, your hair is so nice." I would return the compliment by telling her how I admired her neatly cropped natural hair (and when I returned to the States, I started wearing a similar style).

Short hair remains a popular style among University of Botswana women. Many of them have kept their hair short since early childhood. Shaving the hair from the heads of babies three to five days after birth is a tradition in many homes. This practice applies to both genders. There is a commonly held belief that at conception, the baby is a foreign body, that is, no one knows the child until it is born. Consequently, the newborn child's hair must be cut, since it is "womb hair" grown while the baby was in the uterus. To cleanse the newborn and to prepare her or him for the new environment, the shorn hair and the umbilical cord are buried together in the ground. The newborn is now considered ready for entry into society.

Throughout life, short hair and shaved heads continue to be associated with cleanliness; hence the prominence of close-cropped natural hairstyles and completely shaved heads among women on campus. Many of my students who wore short hair preferred it because they viewed it as being tidy, convenient, manageable, less expensive, cool in the intense heat of summer, and smart looking.

Completely shaving the head as a sign of bereavement for a parent or husband is also practiced in many areas of the country. The custom applies to both male and female children. The exception is the last born child, who will have her or his head shaved a year after the death of the relative. This practice, I was told, is a sign of piety.

Late in the spring, I missed seeing Botho Thobega, our departmental secretary. Then one day she appeared with a shaved head. When I made some comment about how trendy she looked, she explained, "My father is late, so I am compelled to honor his memory by shaving my head." But all students were not as loyal to upholding traditions as Botho. One student commenting on hair and childbirth stated, "I think the tradition of a women who has just given birth having to cut her hair should be dismissed."

On a number of occasions I found myself interrogating an anthropologist, Aylena Segobye, about the diverse hair phenomena I was observing. She said to me, "You know, some Botswana women are shying away from such natural hairstyles as short hair, naturals, dreadlocks, and braids because of the perception that relaxed hair is more attractive and sophisticated. She explained how wearing scarves was associated with being a domestic; the glitzier the hairdo, the more professional the appearance was perceived to be. "As for me, I love all the natural styles," she added.

Unlike many African-American women who visit the beauty salon as frequently as every week or two, women in Botswana, I learned, more typically visit once a month or only for special occasions. Hairdressing is almost the exclusive domain of women, though male expatriate hairstylists from neighboring Zimbabwe, South Africa, and as far away as Germany can be found in some beauty salons. In the capital city, Gaborone, there are beauty salons to meet every need and budget. At the high end are very elegant, Western-style unisex salons with names like Silver Scissors and the Health and Beauty Center where the customer may sip a glass of champagne or a cup of tea while her hair is being done. There are also salons in the city's two five-star hotels.

The traditional hairdressers have thriving businesses because they go to the customer. They usually have no set prices, but they do have the manual dexterity and patience required to execute the many elaborate and time-consuming hairstyles. They view hair as a medium for creative expression and contentedly endure what otherwise would be a long, arduous task.

Generalizations cannot be made about "African" hairstyles or practices. Africa is a vast continent, the second largest in the world. The people who inhabit it are from divergent backgrounds, and differ physically, culturally, and linguistically. Unlike the way black Americans sometimes generalize about Africans, Africans make fine distinctions about African Americans.

One of my colleagues, Laloba, a fifty-something Botswana mother, sported dreadlocks; her twenty-something daughter also wore this style. Laloba said that her adult son referred to her and his sister as "the mop heads." The English majors in my class were just about split in their opinion: some liked the locks; others regarded them as untidy. But they did see an African connection to "dreadlocks," most of them citing the example of Emperor Haile Selassie I of Ethiopia and the Rastafarian doctrine, which in part commands followers to never comb or cut their hair.

The most interesting thing that I learned about Botswana women was the ways that they found to straighten their hair. One method was to heat smooth stones in the sun or fire and move them quickly down the strands of the hair to remove the kinks and flatten the mane. This procedure was repeated until the entire head had been covered. I imagined the women searching the dry Arizona-like terrain for stones of the required size and surface and placing the stones out in lines under the intense midday sun.

A simple bar of Sunlight brand soap, imported from South Africa, was the forerunner to setting lotion. I found out that in some places in the "bush" it is still used for this purpose. Even today, students (including some males) admit to using Sunlight to style their hair. The bar of soap would be worked into a lather and then applied to the wet hair. The hair is styled while the lather is still foaming. Then a scarf is tied tightly around the hair to keep it in place. Once the scarf is removed, the dried hair has a straight yet crinkly texture. A "konk"-like substance was also mentioned to have been used at one time to achieve the smooth, straight look. It is apparent that Western culture has infiltrated Botswana, as it has other countries in Africa. Colonial administrators, missionaries, and more recently the expanding empire of the mass communication media have brought changes in the ways people view themselves.

Although at first glance it could have been a black university campus anywhere, on closer look the University of Botswana seemed distinctive to me because the women students experimented with a broad range of hairstyles without losing touch with their indigenous culture: one day long, the next day short, the next day gone, their changing hairstyles still deeply rooted in their own traditions.

BIG MAMA SAYS:

If a bird gets some of your hair and puts it in his nest, you're a goner.

HEAD TO THE SKY

In Salvador de Bahia, Brazil, in preparation for initiation into the African-Brazilian religion Condomble, initiates have their heads shaved, and white patterns are painted on the head to represent a specific orisha. Orishas are spirits who are the go-between between the person and the Creator. This pattern on the head not only shows which orisha guides them but strengthens their connection to that spirit during this period. So lots of times in Bahia, following their period of reclusion during initiation, you see beautiful, bald woman walking the streets.

—Daniel Minter, visual artist

CROWNING GLORIES: HAIR, HEAD, STYLE,
AND SUBSTANCE IN YORUBA CULTURE

Photos and text by Henry John Drewal

Among Yoruba-speaking peoples of West Africa, the head and its adornment
are central to all cultural life, thought, and practice. The head (*ori*) has two parts—
the outer physical head (*ori ode*) and the inner, spiritual head (*ori inu*). The inner
head is the site of a person's personality, character, individuality, and destiny—it is
what a person chooses from the otherworld before coming to the world. At birth,
Yoruba carefully record the conditions of arrival, watching for signs of the identity
and destiny of the newborn. Such signs are known as *amutorunwaye,* "signs
brought from the other world to the world." They can be seen in the way a child is
born—head first, feet first, in the caul, with a full head of hair, and so on. These
help to determine from whence the child comes. There are three possibilities—
from the mother's lineage, from the father's lineage, or from a divinity (*orisa*). A
child born through the intercession of the divinity of the sea, Olokun, arrives with
a thick crown of hair on its head and is known as Omolokun, "Child of Olokun."
Such a joyous occasion is celebrated in song, which translates to:

Children of the sea with shells on their heads
Rulers today, rulers tomorrow, rulers forever
Fire on the head that water quenches

The child's thick, tightly woven, spiraling hair is likened to a crown of sea
shells. Such hair marks the child as special, divinely born and a future devotee of
Olokun and water spirits generally. Omolokun children are closely related to
other special children born with thick hair who are called Dada. Such children,
because of their relationship to the sacred realm, must be treated in special ways
in order to encourage them to remain in the world rather than leave early to join
spirit companions in the otherworld.

Ceremonies involving the hair must be performed for Dada children. At a
certain time, determined by consultation with an Ifa divination priest, the parents must arrange to have the hair shaved off in a private rite involving prayers,
blessings, and offerings. The soothing, cooling, and healing fluid from a snail is
rubbed on the head and hair to pacify the deity of Dada children.

Bayanni, the older sister of the thunder god, Shango, was known to have long locks of coiled hair that are represented in her sculptures as braids of cowrie shells. Dada-Bayanni children are said to be peace-loving, and a song says, "Dada-Bayanni cannot fight, but she has a younger brother who certainly can!" Since cowries have been the currency since ancient times, the praise name for her hair is *alade owo jinijini,* "owner of crown of money that sounds jinijini [the

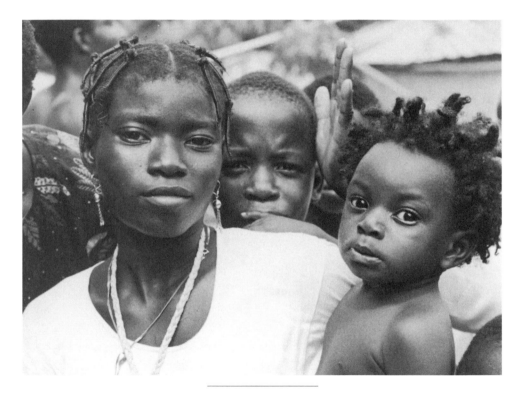

A baby with Dada hair.

sound of cowries strung together]." After cutting, the hair is kept in a special place, and a large celebration is held to honor the child and its auspicious birth, which portends wealth and good fortune.

In the photograph, the sister who holds her Dada brother wears the hairstyle known as "center-parting with one-elbow" named for its primary features—a part down the center of the head, and braids wrapped in thread with one twist or elbow *(esun kan)* near the base.

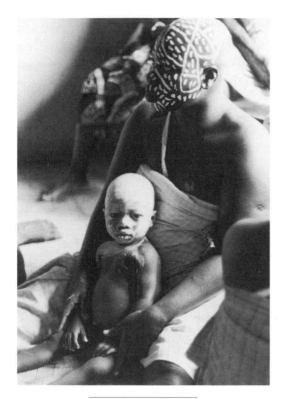

*The patterns painted on this
woman's head are symbolic of the gods.*

Thus the hair that one brings to the world at birth can be a sign that helps to shape a person's life, and the lives of those who live with and love that person, in profound ways.

Yoruba hairstylists/artists, known as *onidiri,* create coiffures of three basic types, defined by technique. The first is *irun biba,* which refers to temporary and less elaborate plaited hair. The second is known as *irun didi* or *olowo*—"done by hand, hand-finished"—in which the hair is parted into intricate designs and woven into braids without thread. The third type is called *irun kiko* or *olowu*—"done with thread"—and came into use about the time of World War II; it involves the wrapping and braiding of the hair using a thread, usually shiny black cotton, or plastic.

COSMOS AND COIFFURES

While the nature of a person's spiritual head is chosen before birth, a person can work on it to ensure that it brings good fortune and positive possibilities. One of the ways is to make it as attractive as possible by embellishing it in myriad ways. Men may keep their hairstyles relatively simple and neat, but women will spend enormous amounts of time creating elaborate coiffures that beautify and enhance their heads in striking ways. A proverb, "May my outer head not disgrace the inner one," reminds Yorubas that one's physical appearance can shape and express as well as reflect one's character in dramatic ways. Let us consider some of the crowning glories—the coiffures and head decorations—that beautify the

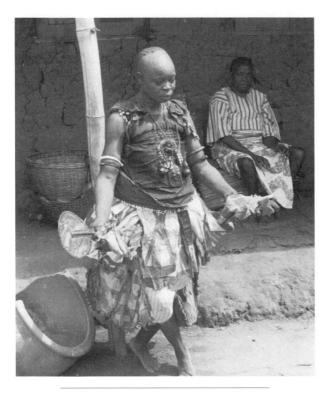

As an invitation to the gods, this priestess has had the hair above her forehead shaven.

heads of Yoruba women showing off their best.

HEADS FIT FOR THE GODS

Persons who dedicate themselves to serving the gods (*orisa*, also known as *orisha*) must have their heads prepared in specific ways to allow them to receive divinity during possession trances. It is during such ceremonies that the gods are said to "mount" their devotees, entering their inner, spiritual heads (*ori inu*) to dwell briefly among the living, bringing blessings and protection. Before this happens, the person must undergo extensive preparation, training, and a final initiation ceremony that involves shaving the head and painting colors and patterns on it that are symbolic of the gods. Such colors and patterns are made with sacred pigments that are at the same time healing, empowering substances—sacred medicines. Priestesses temporarily remove the initiate's hair, which is later allowed to grow back in a kind of tuft known as *osu* on the top of the head, where substances have been placed. Such procedures transform the person's life to one of devotion to the gods. It is a kind of rebirth, the start of a new life. The tuft of hair (or special hairstyle) marks this transformation.

For example, a priestess of the thunder god Shango dances in her god's honor. She wears a skirt of many layers of fabric that swirl on the air as she spins. Note her dramatic coiffure done in special *kolese* style—the hair above her forehead has been shaved off to reveal a broad swelling surface—perhaps a reference to the moment of her initiation, when her head was completely shaved. Her hairstyle evokes the Yoruba metaphor of possession trance, for they say that the head "swells" *(wu)* when the gods come down. At the back of her head, braids have been wrapped and tied to cover her spiritual tuft, the spot where sacred medicines were placed at her initiation. While we no longer see the tuft, her dramatic coiffure announces her priesthood to all, and her capacity to embody Shango during trance dances. Male possession priests of Shango are also known as Iyawo

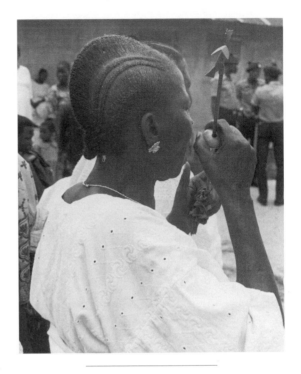

This style represents the close bond between a mother and her children

Shango, "brides of Shango." During festivals they wear their hair in a female style, usually *kolese,* perhaps because it is the easiest to weave. *Kolese,* "without legs," refers to the hair weaving that begins in the front and ends at the back, without any braids that stand up. It is regarded as a simple and quick style to make, so mothers in a hurry use it for their children on school days.

BRAIDS AND BEADS IN HONOR OF A QUEEN

In the ancient Yoruba city of Owo, the community annually celebrates a famous queen, Oronsen, who helped them conquer their enemies. Oronsen was renowned for her beauty, wealth, and influence, and most especially for her extraordinary hair.

During Oronsen's festival, called Igogo, no one is permitted to cover her or his head with anything, whether headties or hats. Young girls dress in their finest beads as signs of wealth and status. With the help of their mothers and sisters they also create multiple elaborate buns of hair to crown their heads, as Queen Oronsen might have done many generations ago. In one such style vertical braids are gathered in a big bun at the top. At the sides and curling in front of the ears are other entwined braids. The style is known as Moremi, in honor of another famous queen (at Ile-Ife), who also helped her people defeat an enemy.

Another wears the *kolese* style with weaving from the front to the back, but

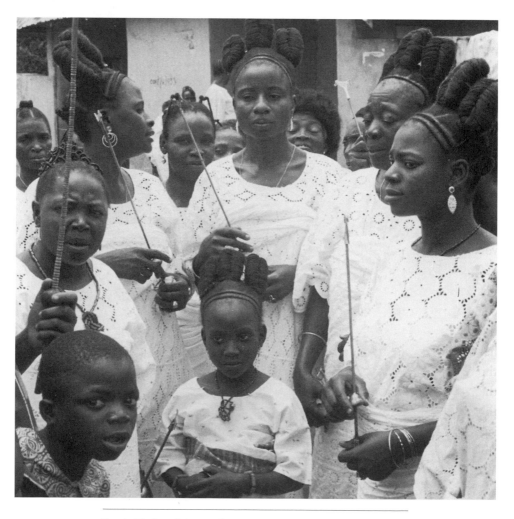

Special hairstyles worn by royal women and girls at a festival.

with a difference—the high "hen's comb" at the center and smaller braids at the sides. The name given to this coiffure evokes the close bond of love between a mother and her children—*arin omo lemi o sun,* "I will rest (be buried) in the midst of my children." In polygamous Yoruba society, the bond between mother and child is usually regarded as stronger than that between father and child. The Yoruba saying, "Mother is gold, father is glass" *(iya ni wura, b aba ni digi),* graphically conveys this idea. This woman, and others at Owo during the Igogo festival, carry small iron staffs with birds on the top—a supreme symbol of the mystical power of women to bring life into the world (and remove it as well). The women strike these staffs with iron rings to provide the rhythms for songs as they process through the town in honor of Queen Oronsen.

Along with many strands of body beads, young girls insert exquisite hair ornaments, pins, jewelry, and combs to highlight their tufts and braids of hair. As they move through the streets of the city, people sing their praises. The sight is wonderful, literally "full of wonder," as the Yoruba would say.

But perhaps the most spectacular hair-

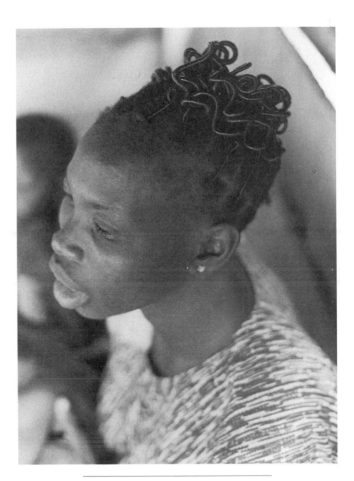

Energtic coils created by wrapping the hair with shiny black thread.

styles are those worn by women of the royal family. They come out elegantly dressed in white lace dresses, holding iron staffs with birds. Their heads are embellished in extraordinary buns that stand up vertically—three across the top of their heads behind one or two rows of low braids that go across their foreheads from ear to ear. Another style worn by women features tall, spiraling braids that come together at the top. This style, "Cocoa House" or Onile Ogogoro, was named in honor of the first skyscraper built in Yorubaland in the city of Ibadan.

At the climax of the Igogo festival comes the Ojomo, king of Ijebu-Owo in Owo City. Shaded under a large umbrella, he walks surrounded by his subjects. He

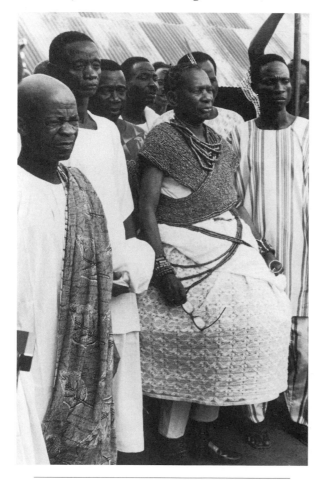

wears a large voluminous hooped skirt, his torso is covered in multiple strands of stone and coral beads, and his hair is braided in female fashion, with parrots' feathers, to commemorate Queen Oronsen.

HAIR THAT SPEAKS

The names of several popular hairstyles either reveal social attitudes or commemorate historical moments. A smiling young mother nurses her child within the family domestic compound. Her elaborate coiffure (and earrings) hint at a coming celebration, perhaps the child-naming ceremony of her infant. Her hairstyle,

To commemorate an ancient brave queen, the king wears a female hairstyle and hoop skirt.

called *panumo*—"Shut your mouth!" or "Keep things secret!"—refers to the dangers and consequences of malicious gossip. This idea is visually invoked in wrapped braids that start at the front and back of the head and meet in the center, like two sealed lips!

HAIR AS HISTORY

Women's coiffures are sometimes represented in Yoruba masquerades performed by men. In one ancestral masquerade (*egungun*) known as Iyawo, "Wife," a hairstyle composed of rounded arches is called "Eko Bridge," to commemorate the elegant structure of the new bridge connecting Lagos Island with mainland Nigeria, completed in 1970. Another style created in January 1970 was called Ogun Pari, "War Has Ended." Five tall arched braids on each side are then tied together to form a circle, commemorating the end of the Nigerian civil war.

In another, equally creative style, the braids of a young Yoruba woman are wrapped in shiny black threads and coiled, curled, and

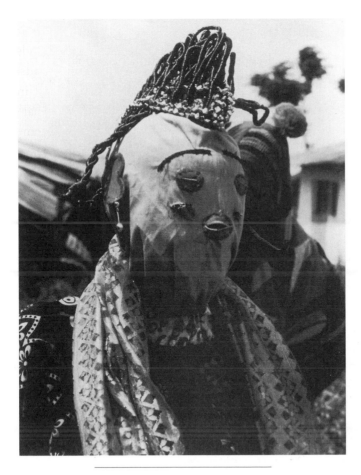

This style was created to commemorate an important Nigerian bridge.

twisted in a complex composition that gives a wonderful sense of energy and movement.

The world of Yoruba women's hairstyles is rich in meaning and breathtaking beauty and inventiveness. As my colleague and friend Olabiyi Yai has said, Yoruba consider their artists to be itinerant persons "engaged in constant departures of creativity." Certainly the hairstylists of Yorubaland are no exception. May we always enjoy their crowning creations. *Ase!*

NO LONGER STRANDED

Idara E. Bassey

I could not help but smile to myself when a brother with a beautiful head full of locks pulled up in the lane next to mine, poised at the wheel of a minivan with a small army of chocolate-colored children. I thought to myself, What caption best fits this picture—Rasta abandons the revolution? How to domesticate your dreadlocked one?

I am a Nigerian-American woman fascinated by locks, and by extension (no pun intended) with the unlimited potential of our hair in its natural state. My uncle, who spent his formative years in Nigeria, was born with hair that grew in dreadlocked fashion naturally. Such children were collectively known as Dada (a reference to the similarity of their hair texture to that commonly seen among the Yoruba, Nigeria's third largest ethnic group, who are concentrated in the southwestern portion of the country). There was a universally held belief that such hair symbolized strength and that the wearer would be blessed with great wealth in the future.

My uncle was among the children that were seen as special; their hair could not be washed or cut until a special ritual ceremony, held at the urging of the parents or other elders. At the time of the ceremony, their hair would be shaved off and normal hair growth would resume. Older children who still had their "locks" were expected to show their "wealth" by distributing gifts (usually sugarcane or cookies) to the other children in the neighborhood who had not been as fortunate. Today, the demands of Nigeria's increasingly urbanized life have all but discouraged individuals from remaining Dada.

After my first year at law school, I shaved off my shoulder-length hair and wore a "box" cut—short on the top and virtually nonexistent on the sides—and fielded an avalanche of negative comments and pointed questions well into my third and final year.

My relatives back home were horrified by my new style. A woman's beauty is attributed to her hair, was the oft-repeated refrain. One aunt or another would initiate the discussion, invariably smoothing down her "coiffed-in-America" weave protectively during the course of the conversation, as if to ensure that whatever brought on my egregious error in judgment was not catching. My Caribbean friends' reactions were no improvement. The Jamaican medical student I was dating at the time greeted my first "post-box" debut with a wan smile.

Many of my African women friends remain caught in a vise: pressured on one side by the feminine ideals promulgated by Western media and on the other by family and tradition. An Ethiopian sister I spoke with admits she has been

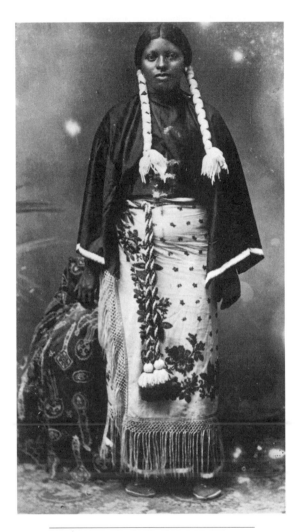

In colonial America, the cultures of Africans and Native Americans got braided through inter-marriage and other encounters. Diana Fletcher, a nineteenth-century black woman, lived with the Kiowa Indian nation.

WESTERN HISTORY COLLECTIONS, UNIVERSITY OF OKLAHOMA LIBRARIES thinking about cutting her hair but fails to do so because her mother would "hate" it. A sister-friend of Nigerian and Haitian descent agonizes over her family's reaction to her double-strand twists. And a former roommate from Tanzania spends all her waking hours with her "hair" on—a synthetic creation mimicking a permed 'do. As Western mass media grows ever more powerful and global, it's hard for women anywhere to maintain their individuality.

Now, several years out of law school, I am cultivating an inner fearlessness. In 1998 I decided to leave my firm and pursue self-employment. My hair reflects the change, moving as it has from shoulder-length braids shaped into a bob to quietly rebellious double-strand twists. In the process, I have become particularly sensitive to the rhythms and the mysteries of my hair, and I am absolutely thrilled with this bold turn of events.

Thoughts of the immaculate locks of the brother speeding away that glorious sunny afternoon still surface from time to time, and I cannot help but wonder, How would he have looked on a horse?

Silver Foxes

as Mama says, "You don't get old bein' no fool." Silver hair, then, is like a glowing medal of honor, conferred upon those who live long, wise, and well. This aura of light framing a warm brown face is a beauty to behold. And let us not forget that even the $100 jar of wrinkle-fighting cream is no match for melanin, which keeps our skin smooth well into our golden years.

A FLASH OF SILVER

In the early 1950s, Joyce Bryant appeared on a bill with Josephine Baker. Knowing she had to do something to distinguish herself, the dark and lovely chanteuse donned a silver dress, silver nails, and a silver floor-length mink. To top it off, she painted her hair silver. Bryant belted out "Love for Sale" and "Drunk with Love"—both hit records, though they were a little too risqué to be played on the radio. But the hair brought the house down.

"I stopped everything!" she told a reporter, who went on to note, "The silver radiator paint she had used (this was before such hair dyes were available) also almost cost her her hair, but it became a trademark."

—"After the Age of Silver," *New York Times*, July 22, 1977

MY SMART GRAY STREAK
Yvonne Durant

"If you make me look good, I'll make you look good." That was my gray hair talking to my face several years ago. I don't think my face was so excited at first. Free of wrinkles, it had 'em guessing for years. But so far the arrangement is working.

It was nearly a decade ago, when I was in my mid-thirties, that I became aware of a gray streak making its way into my dark brown hair. After leaving a smudge of the black mascara I'd used to hide a couple of pushy gray strands on the chin of a boyfriend, I decided to let my hair be. Perhaps I felt more daring because I was living in Milan, Italy, away from all the folks who knew me when. In that country, it seems that every man of a certain age sports exquisite silver-gray hair. Women, on the other hand, fight it all the way; they remain miraculously blonde, brunette, or black-haired well into their later years. So letting my true colors show there proved to be an unexpectedly bold feat.

As I moved through the piazzas, people would

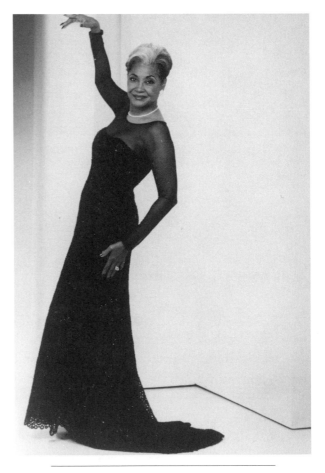

Nancy Wilson set the elegant chanteuse standard in the late 1950s and maintains it today.

CHARLES WILLIAM BUSH

stare at me, as they normally did at someone obviously not Italian. Still, the combination of brown skin and gray streak seemed to give me some celebrity. I took it in stride, strolling up Monte Napoleone, enjoying my weekly visit to the spot where the chic shop chic. The sleek fit of my slacks and my wrinkle-free skin set against my "white hairs," as the row of women vendors called them, confused many. Who knows how many lire were won or lost guessing my age?

Youth. So many people assumed that you trade it away when you choose to stop coloring your hair. I don't agree. There is an added crispness to the texture of gray hair that can make it more challenging to manage; yet I believe that that is offset by the cool air of grace gray evokes. My mother has been gray for as long as I can remember, and I've always admired her aura of sophistication, which I'm sure is enhanced by her fabulous hair. This has everything to do with beauty and nothing to do with age. But age is a factor. . . .

"Are you mother and daughter?" the hostess asked me and my sister as we sat in an East Side restaurant in New York City one day, a few years ago.

I answered the question with an attitude, because the woman looked at me when she said "mother."

"She's my sister," I responded. "Do I look as if I have a forty-one-year-old daughter?" The hostess was horrified. But my sister, Yvette, was initially amused, and then later annoyed that the whole restaurant now knew her age. Did I mention that Yvette is my twin?

Girlfriends mean well in their own way. They scold me because they say I make myself look older. For the longest time, only one friend gave me a clear-cut compliment; she admired my confidence. It took me some time to realize that in letting my hair evolve naturally, I've become an innocent tattletale. If I'm the one woman in the room with gray hair and all the others are more or less my age, one can safely assume that someone is coloring her hair—and it's not me.

What do the gentlemen think? Gray makes them look twice. Their eyes dance between the face and the hair, and they see something that doesn't add up. "If you're comfortable with it, I'm comfortable," said one friend. "I like the honesty," he added. Young guys seem to think they've done me a favor by acknowledging my presence. "Surprised I'm talking to you?" one asked. "Not at all," I answered. Another pointed me out to his friends as I walked by, "See, that's my type of woman: She's old enough. You can tell she has wisdom." Wisdom? I'll take it.

Some men, usually older, make eye contact and give me a nod of approval. I

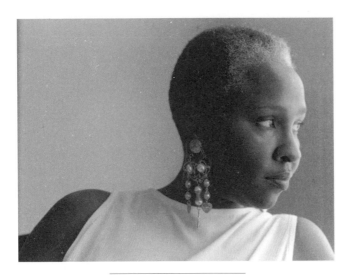

Brenda, Philadelphia, 1993.

BILL GASKINS

thank them with a knowing smile. What they see in me is a woman young enough but not too young, with a certain maturity. I'm safe for fragile egos.

My credibility has increased in recent years. My hair seems to have upped my IQ considerably; at least that's how I'm treated. When I talk, people listen. They probably always have, but now they really seem to want to know what I think. Physically, I have become the woman I will be. I've been waiting for my forties. My body has been kind to me, and my hair did just the right thing. I have been kind to myself by welcoming what age has brought me.

I'm the twin with the gray hair. I'm the woman with the gray streak. I'm the daughter who's almost as gray as her parents. I'm the glamorous girlfriend. Glamorous? I'll take it.

BIG MAMA SAYS

If you pull a white hair, seven more will come to its funeral.

ATTITUDE AT SEVENTY-FIVE
Naomi Long Madgett

In this recurring dream I am Tina Turner
flinging my wild wig at the world,
strut-stomping across the stage
on miniskirted gams ageless and untamed,

completely in command and belting out
my song,
What's Time Got to Do With It!

IN HER HAIR
S. Pearl Sharp

After completing her daily gardening and a small lunch, Julia Lyons went to her room, pulled back the embroidered white cotton sheets, and laid down ninety-one years of living. She refused to get up.

Granddaughters and nieces scurried up and down the carpeted stairs, a chorus of whispers dressed in a collective frown. Julia, her arms crossed over her chest and her eyes closed, brusquely dismissed the doctor they summoned, stating firmly, "I need some quiet time. I'm thinking."

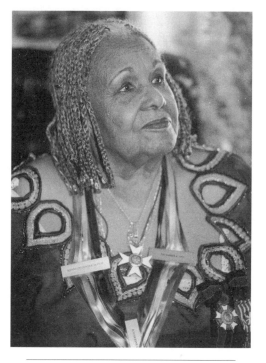

Pioneering African-American modern dancer Katherine Dunham in 1992 at 82 years old.

ODELL MITCHELL JR.

On the third morning she announced she would, at last, meet her great-great-granddaughter in a few hours. The family matriarch was immediately declared delirious, and those ominous "You better come right away" calls went out to points across Ohio.

But there was no answer at my house. Hours earlier we had beat the dawn to Highway 42, a five-hour drive ahead of us. I was eight months old, and already knew it would be disrespectful to make an elder look like a liar. I arrived at the venerable house exactly as Julia had predicted.

There was a hushed sparkle in the room. Blood, five generations deep, seeing survival in each other's eyes. The born free, colored, Negro, soon-to-be-black, all here. Blood. Laughing, anticipating, humming. And then, with mutual awe, the new-life eyes and the ancient eyes beheld each other.

After a few moments my great-great-grandmother motioned for me to be taken away. As I was lifted from her arms, she held on a moment longer, her crinkled fingers molding themselves around my small head.

"She's just been waiting to see this baby," the women proclaimed. As they elaborated on the splendor of the waiting (as if this eternal ritual was something new), Julia smiled and, without their permission, went off to see what her God was doing for lunch.

Don't look for her power
in the eyes
or the thighs,
Look in her hair . . .
There are secrets birthing there . . .

Twelve X one. The story, repeated often by my mother, was forgotten until strands of silver began to dance on the top of my head. "Premature," they were labeled. I didn't think so. I was twelve years old, and felt they were right on time for something, I just wasn't sure what. I imagined they grew exactly where great-great-grandmama what's-her-name had touched me.

Twelve X two. Alone in the city of ten million, missing those Friday nights when three generations of black women would "scratch hair." Sitting on the floor, warm between my grandmother Nana's legs as she whisked the bristles across my scalp, finding a way through the terrible thickness, yellow electricity flying from the end of the brush. And Bunny, my mother, standing behind us with Nana's favorite thick black plastic comb. She would scratch her mother's scalp and ask, "Don't you know how to say stop? Enough!?" Nana never did. (Nana, who only cut hair on the new moon. It was one of our games—Bunny pretending to shame Nana into an ending word and Nana pretending she couldn't hear.) I supplied the giggles. When I grew tall enough, the honor of scratching Nana's head was sometimes handed over to me. I would come to understand it as the way a woman who was not given to affection allowed herself to be touched.

Twelve X three. The silver strands from a congregation, giving me an ID tag in the land of illusion.

"How does your hairdresser do that?" they ask.

"She takes her time," I answer with a sly smile.

"OK, we'll just dye it." This from a television director who doesn't see me, only some hair with a problem.

"Dye it and die," I respond. Because now I recognize that nothing really bad ever happens to me. I am powerfully protected by the hand that carried my blood and blessed my head.

Look in her hair
There are secrets birthing there . . .

My hair is Matt's* transmitter, broadcasting the latest news. I learn to read my state of health through it. Are there other things it wants to tell me? How do I listen?

The dot of gray becomes a patch,
becomes a stream . . .

Bunny is dying. This message comes to me one morning when I comb my hair and discover a naked circle of scalp the size of a silver dollar. My stomach churns. Chemotherapy treatments have taken my mother's hair, and she is taking mine with her. Must we be so damn connected?

Six weeks after she dies, as I refocus on my own life, I ponder damage control for the bald spot. But a soft fuzziness meets my fingers, the circle no longer naked. She has given me back to myself.

Twelve X four. "Learn to grow old gracefully," Nana had always admonished. And finally I hear her.

"Don't dye it, don't pull it out. These are blessings and messages from your ancestors," I insist, encouraging sistas who are afraid of their gray. "Don't mess with the message!" And I rejoice with each sister who resists the white American quest to be forever young.

Apart from my own life, what makes me believe my words? Perhaps it is Mama Pansa, a slave on the run in Suriname, who braided rice seeds in her hair so her people would have food to plant where they resettled. Perhaps it is friends talking about the intensity with which they perceive things since letting their hair grow into dreadlocks—picking up stuff they could never sense before.

---

*Maat was an ancient Egyptian deity whose hair rose like antennae from the top of her head.

Don't look for her power
in the eyes
or the thighs,
Look in her hair . . .

I often marvel at the power my great-great-ancestor had, the power to embrace an infant with a circle of protection that lasts a lifetime. My job, I've come to understand, is to protect and give honor to the blessing. Do not test this gift unduly, do not molest it, do not go out and act a fool on the assumption of divine protection.

The hair Julia touched has become its own diva. I am simply the housekeeper, listening to the messages, reading the waves, dancing to the songs my great-great-grandmama planted there.

HOMAGE TO MY HAIR
Lucille Clifton

when i feel her jump up and dance
i hear the music! my God
i'm talking about my nappy hair!
she is a challenge to your hand
black man,
she is as tasty on your tongue as good greens
black man,
she can touch your mind
with her electric fingers and
the grayer she do get, good God
the blacker she do be!

SOMETHING'S LOST IN LIVING EVERY DAY
Leatha Simmons Mitchell

As I enter my seventh decade, my hair is long, dry, and fragile, with silver

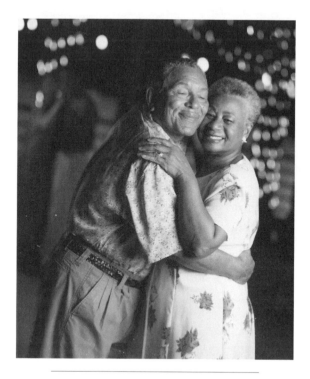

"When we're out together dancing cheek to cheek."

STEVE CHENN/CORBIS

stripes shooting through the front and temples like the plumage of an exotic bird. When wet, its crinkly waves reach below my shoulder blades. Despite bouts of unruliness, it has been the source of lifelong sensuous delight. A marvelous medium for experimentation, my hair is a magical extension of myself. But now my delight is tinged with apprehension as each morning I pull wads of hair from my brush. Where hairdressers once thinned my hair to achieve various styles, my tresses now require careful combing to conceal bare patches on my crown.

At times I feel seized by sadness, unprepared to lose my hair, my friend. I know I'm not alone. I am reminded of other women who in the past have confided in me about the trauma of their hair loss. I gave them glib advice about taking vitamins (especially inositol), scalp massage, and the bits and scraps I'd picked up from women's magazines. I shored these sisters up with reassurances, never truly fathoming what this loss must have meant to them. Now I realize that the underlying feeling is one of shame and sorrow. A bald head, unless a woman chooses it deliberately, is humiliating.

Throughout the ages, shaving a woman's head in many cultures has been a way of punishing her for adultery or prostitution. Neither wholly utilitarian nor completely decorative, hair offers a woman simple comfort. Mine is still thick enough that, when rolled into a bun, it cushions my neck as I lie down. Running my fingers through it, in countless repetitions, is a meditative, soothing ritual that eases the grip of despair and stimulates tender memories.

My very first hair memory is of being sixteen months old, kicking and screaming during shampoo sessions. I only relaxed in the hands of my mother's mother. In the few black-and-white photographs we have of her, her marcelled tresses are startling black against white skin, which I remember as being the color of freshly churned butter. To shield my eyes from the suds, she stretched me out over her lap, positioned a basin on the floor, and gently poured pitchers of water over my scalp to rinse away the lather. Her lap was soft, her hand stroking my forehead, gentle. Love flowed with the water.

When I was school age, picture days were the most dreaded of all. My mother would wash my hair the night before and braid it in knuckle-knocking braids that shrank until they were barely shoulder-length. Since it was winter, I had to wear a woolen cap, which flattened my hair to my head like a helmet. Invariably, the photographer's flash captured me at my worst. Even today, depending on my mood, I either cringe or laugh out loud at these portraits in which I am a human octopus, the ends of my wet braids curled on my shoulders like bizarre tentacles.

On occasion, Mama would roll my hair up on curlers made of strips of torn paper bags, twisting the ends. The result was fat, black, sausage-shaped curls on which an outsize, floppy bow would be affixed. Several times she gave me a Toni, the early home permanent touted on radio and billboards with ads asking the question, "Which twin has the Toni?" But the ammonia in the product left the house smelling like the barn of a careless farmer, and the results hardly seemed worth it. On rare occasions when my father was away from home, she would sneak out the straightening comb, and I'd be her Indian maiden for a few days until my hair reverted to its natural crinkles.

Still, I never criticized my mother for making me look at best hopelessly old-fashioned, and at worst ridiculous—especially since she seemed to think that her touch only enhanced me. In her country-hewn aesthetic, beauty was defined by order. She favored things neatly tied down and bundled, whether hay or hair. And she preferred them polished and oiled, whether furniture or faces.

In my early teens, summer spelled escape from the painful shyness I felt in school. In summer, we were no longer housebound by Pennsylvania's interminable winters. The odors of coal-burning fires, bean stews, and wet clothing gave way to the blissful scents of apple blossoms and peaches cooking in preparation for the canning jars. There was a fringe of forest behind our house and a creek. My brothers and I spent those precious few months gathering wild black-berries and catching butterflies. I ran everywhere, exhilarated by the feel of my hair whipping against my face. When the day was near done, I would sometimes stand before my bedroom mirror with the western sun washing over my body. It highlighted the fiery red strands in my hair, and I felt goddess beautiful.

Still, the boredom of our borough of slightly less than a thousand souls made me hunger for greater adventures. Since I had grown too tall to be a jockey, my aspirations wavered from writing true confession stories to joining a nunnery. In books, I gravitated toward Greek myths about powerful goddesses who lived free in their sylvan abodes. When I put the books down, I spent hours imagining my-self in exotic places with someone who adored me and my wild, abundant hair.

My adolescent yearning matured into a desire for a sense of shared adventure with another. And while no man with whom I've been intimate has found special delight in my mane, occasionally, at the subway or in a carry-out restaurant, a younger man will comment, "I like your hair like that," meaning loose and free. Or sometimes when I visit another office at the university where I work, a man my age will say, "I remembered you because of your hair." Descending the very long escalators at Dupont Circle in Washington, D.C., my hair blowing in the updrafts, I may catch the eye of a man rising toward the light, who smiles at me. The compliments, both silent and spoken, sustain me, especially as I say good-bye each day to a little part of myself.

I first discovered the problem in 1993 in South Carolina during a family re-union. After sitting in the languid Kiawah Island surf until dusk, I returned to my hotel room to locate and doctor my mosquito bites with the aid of the bath-room's three-way mirror. Looking into it at a certain angle, I was shocked to dis-cover a bald spot in the center of my scalp.

For several days I obsessed over it. Yes, there had been five years of nonstop stress: two breast surgeries for benign cysts; my parents' divorce after fifty-five years; my mother-in-law's passing; my beloved father's slow death from lym-phatic cancer; a rash of serious illnesses around the office. There was also marital and mothering stress; my bonus baby was born when I was forty-six.

Still, I resolved that I would be sensible. I would try to find the cause and, where I could, correct it. I began to choose products without sodium laurel sul-fate, a sudsing agent found in most shampoos that has been implicated in hair loss, and perhaps even in cancer. But there was little I could do about fibromyalgia, a painful multifaceted disease that I've been battling for over seven years, and which is also associated with hair loss. I had to accept that genetics, too, probably played a part. Family reunions confirm that female relatives of my generation have seldom retained the thick, shining hair depicted in their photographs of earlier years. And I recall my paternal grandmother, whose waist-length hair, as she aged, resembled thin, silken ribbons.

Even in that moment when I discovered the bare spot, however, I decided that I would not relentlessly seek a cure. I would consider what could be done, but I would not allow hair loss to define me. I learned to set limits through watching a dear friend passionately grieve the loss of her own hair, trying product after product without success. Sometimes she retires from the battle, only to have her hopes stirred again by the latest potion.

Hair is important, but I don't regard it with the gravity I do those body parts that require the annual scrutiny of pelvic exams, mammograms, and glaucoma screenings. Hair doesn't warrant obsession. So I try not to think about it except at those moments when I'm actually grooming it.

Luckily, I've come to this stage of my life prepared. Twenty years ago, a friend gave me *Creative Visualization* by Shakti Gawain. The book was a portal to universal consciousness and the beginning of a spiritual odyssey that freed me from the sense of mourning that pervades the lives of many of my pre-menopausal, menopausal, and postmenopausal friends. However, I still regret what is happening. Like most women of my age, I've probably lavished more money, time, energy, and care on my hair than on any other part of my anatomy. I've spent a queen's ransom on pH-balanced shampoos, herbal conditioners, holding sprays, spritzers, detanglers, defrizzers, gels, creams, oils, dyes, scrunchees, curlers, headbands, hats, relaxers, wide-toothed combs, natural bristle brushes, blow-dryers, and vitamins—not to mention salon bills.

Even so, caring for my hair has been more of a love affair than a chore. When I get up at night to go to the bathroom, I glance in the mirror, carefully smoothing my hair down. I may steal a glimpse in a store window or before a subway train picks up speed, admiring this hair that I inherited as a gift. It is a better one than the arthritis or the allergies, but it is still a gift. I cherish it, even as I pull it from my brush.

TWO GENERATIONS

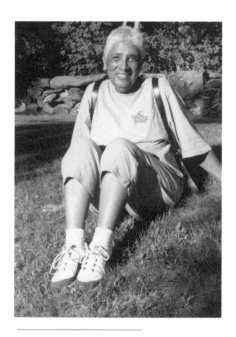

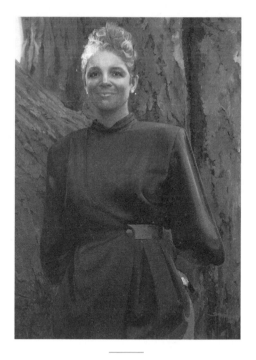

Camille.
Oil on linen, 1990.

PORTRAIT BY SIMMIE KNOX

Catherine C. Hanks
pauses during a hike in
Massachusetts, July 2000.
Born in 1922, she is the
mother of four
children, Camille Cosby
(shown above right),
Guy A. Hanks, Eric
Hanks, and René
Hanks, as well as nine
grandchildren and four
great-grandchildren.
Exercising regularly to
stay fit, Catherine Hanks
has scaled the Swiss Alps
and hiked along the
Appalachian trail.

PHOTO ERIC HANKS

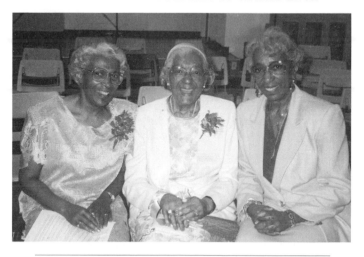

Two more generations. Helen E. Moore, age 93, flanked by her
daughters Anita Moore Hackney (right) and Martha Moore
Mundell at the wedding of Mundell's daughter.

ANITA HACKNEY COLLECTION

THOUGHTS TAKE FLIGHT

A woman sits on the ground in her backyard among fluffy coronas that look like the soft gray fuzz on her head. As she gazes at the white puffs that just days ago were yellow dandelion heads—seeds attached by slender fibers to radiating hairs (perfect flying machines)—she realizes that both the dandelions and her body are being prepared for release. "How wonderful and how right," she thinks. "We are gently disintegrating so that we can fly off in all directions, descend, take root, and blossom again."

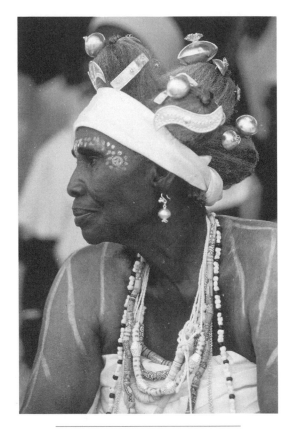

Fante priestess at annual Fetu Afahye Festival at the chief's palace in Winneba, Ghana.

PHOTO ANGELA FISHER/CAROL BECKWITH

SHE WHO MIRRORS ME

Ruby Dee

Sometimes the elements that make up a life are so scary or suddenly depressing, magical, overwhelming, or sinister that more than breathing comes hard. Speaking of age, I am reminded of the time when I was preparing for the role of Mother Abagail in *The Stand*. Mother Abagail was 106 years old. I had stopped coloring my hair, hoping to help shorten the three-hour makeup job required for a younger actor like me. During the transition, I wore wigs most of the time.

One night, however, while scurrying from activity to activity, the hair rose all over my body as, in the half-light, I encountered a white-haired creature coming directly at me, mouth open and garments flapping. I stopped. The creature stopped. I turned, the creature turned. It was I! I was looking at myself in the mirror that had been installed on the landing in my absence; I'd ordered it long ago and had forgotten about it.

I saw something in that mirror that I had never seen before. I had become all the old ladies I'd ever seen, written, or read about. Witch, angel, hag, grandmother sitting in rocking chairs or porches, crone, senior citizen, bag lady, Elder of the Tribe. The staring apparition began to giggle, so I giggled too, and bounded down the steps to tell Ossie of the fright I'd seen, and how that old lady in the mirror had scared the hell out of me. We laughed and laughed and then I cried—cried because here I was, living longer than my grandmother, my mother, all my aunts, father, brother, sister! I cried also with joy because that old lady in the mirror and I—we'd made it!

How lucky, how marvelous, not to be dead yet. Fear. Oh, it will all soon be over. Death. Let it do its own advertising, I thought. I'll spend those last few minutes kicking up my heels, writing about the contradictions, absurdities, joys, and responsibilities of living long, and let the permanently horizontal mode and intimations of mortality take care of themselves.

GRAY STRANDS
Naomi Long Madgett

1 Badge of trial
and triumph:
it is mine, I have
earned it.
I wear it proudly

2 There is nothing
more lovely
than silver framing
a face
of old ebony.

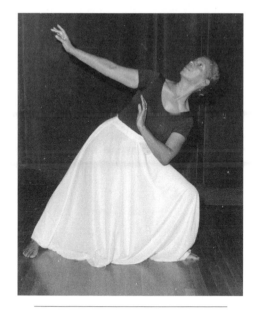

Nina Butts, director of the dance program at Hampton University, started teaching there in 1960. She still performs in the department's annual spring concerts.

PHOTO REUBEN BURRELL

Locks and Keys

When we are comfortable with ourselves, every day is a good hair day. This journey to self-acceptance can be a long one, with many twists and turns, but for every sister there is a solution.

BRAIDED SATURN RING ASTOUNDS SCIENTISTS

"It defies the laws of orbital mechanics as I understand them but two components of the fifth ring out are braided," said Dr. Bradford Smith of the rings of Saturn, as reported in the November 13, 1980, *Washington Post*. Smith—a University of Arizona scientist—and several of his colleagues were gathered at the Jet Propulsion Laboratory in Pasadena, California, studying photographs transmitted back to Earth from the spacecraft *Vogager*. "If the distribution of these braids is uniform around the entire ring," Smith observed, "then there are as many as 1,000 braids in the ring."

Not only was the fifth ring in braids, Smith said, but the 500-mile-long plaits appeared to have kinks in them. As bizarre as the braids are, Smith added, the kinks are even more bizarre: "If you look closely, you see abrupt bends in the braids, as if somebody took the surface and bent it. I don't even pretend to understand what this means."

DON'T EVEN PRETEND (THE SATURN POEM)
Peter Harris

Saturn's rings was all nappy
spread out from her head
like she just woke up
took a shower & ain't dried them yet
dreadlocks

cluttered with moons/meteors/mysteries
so God, She said:

"girl . . . now you know
I can't let you be orbiting round me
looking like that, suppose we have company.
what they gon think of me?"

God took off from work
unscrewed Her Afro
Sheen jar
washed her comb &
pick
sat under constella-
tions
& told Saturn to sit
on the space
between Her legs.
"honey, I got to plait
your rings
even if I miss a day's
pay."

so God got to corn-
rowing Saturn's rings

ain't nothing more
coaxing than God's
hands
spreading each ring
into 3 strands
sifting though rocks

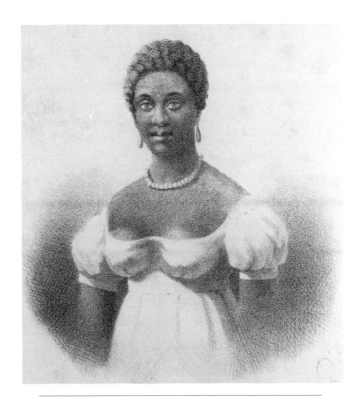

Phillis Wheatley sans headkerchief. An eighteenth-century
French artist depicted the sable poet of Boston in an Empire
gown and elegant, fuzzy coif.

SCHOMBURG CENTER FOR
RESEARCH IN BLACK CULTURE

that was worlds eons ago
she finger Afro Sheen down the part
softening scalp/loosening crusty moons
stuck in orbit
She start humming Nina Simone
while threading wisdom down each row

"here comes the sun
little darlin
here comes the sun . . ."

hands so knowing
they tug/twist/twirl those knotty rings
& Saturn don't whine
just listen to the lyrics
& feel tight lightness
creeping along her scalp
down her back into infinity
Saturn close her eyes
& feel peaceful
like when God rubbed Her palms
for the sixth time & rolled rings
from the swirls in the fingerprints
of each hand

"here comes the sun
little darlin
here comes the sun . . ."

God weave bright beads, baubles & shells
yellow curves/purple swoops/blue loops
decorate the arcs spreading now

like the stiff necklaces
around the throats of Masai sisters

"there child, I'm finished!
my my, you look like a magic pinwheel gracing space.
here, look in my corona
& see how pretty you are."

God hum & sigh
She got to rest these few more hours
work again tomorrow
smiling early from the east
glinting off Saturn's rings
like a fawn darting quenched from a water hole
back into the forest.

IN THE KITCHEN
Jewelle Gomez

When I was a girl, the back of your head, which narrowed softly into your neck, was referred to disdainfully as "the kitchen." I don't know why. There, at the tender slope of the head, the natural texture of our hair seemed to fight for its life. The "naps" that every parent taught us to hate, sprang to life, curling tightly around themselves into small, individual beads, defying the curses of mothers, beauticians, chemicals, and hot combs. It was decades before I believed that those tender naps were not an insult to beauty but a natural part of it. Between then and now I've saved snapshots of the many colored girls who suffered the same assaults on the kitchen as I and survived.

1 "How her mother let her leave the house like that?" The eyes of neighborhood mothers spoke more loudly than any words they dared to say. And the young woman with the short Afro walked down Tremont Street in the south end of Boston as if she were strolling the bank of the Niger River. Any time I saw her in our mixed, working-class neighborhood in

the early 1960s, my gaze was riveted to the spectacle of openly displayed naps coiffed into a modest yet regal crown.

"Conk," "do," "process," "permanent," "relaxer" were code words for "I am ugly unless I look like white people." And she was the first person I ever saw who had a real alternative. All I knew about her was her name: Gilda. To me, at age twelve, she was a visitor from another galaxy where little colored girls didn't have to be tortured every two weeks. Probably only sixteen, she wore ordinary clothes, talked ordinary talk. But she was an antidote to every self-hating remark I'd heard from kids and adults in my neighborhood, in my beauty parlour, on my television, in my head.

Deep inside, even then, I held the secret knowledge that I would grow up to be a lover of women. Without ever having heard a word spoken I also understood I would be looked upon with scorn, just as Gilda was, if the neighbors knew my secret. Without her knowledge, that young woman walking serenely, defiantly through my neighborhood was leading me toward my own liberation from the tyranny of straight hair and the deep love of my natural self. And how did her mother let her leave the house like that?

2 Standing in my stepmother Henrietta's kitchen, I'm clutching the hot curling iron. One of her shiny curls clings to the smoking rod. I tug firmly as she's taught me to. The curl pulls away from her head. Completely. It is a burnt thing on the iron,

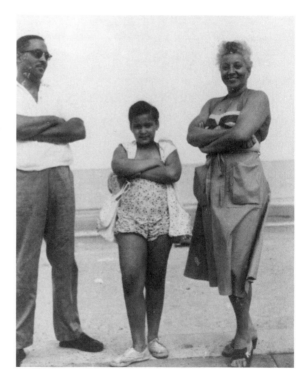

Jewelle Gomez and her grandmother Lydia,
back in the day.

leaving an empty space in my stepmother's going-to-work hairdo. I gulp in terror; she laughs, grabs the iron and the scissors, and takes over.

3 Even though I loved singer Jackie Wilson, I couldn't date boys who straightened their hair. I once tried a slow dance with a neighborhood guy and I recoiled when my hand touched his slicked-down hair. It felt dead, as if it'd been preserved in formaldehyde. I was even more out of step, since all the girls seemed to love it. I wondered then if that really confirmed my future as a lesbian.

4 I have several photographs of my no-cookie-baking grandmother Lydia at the beach. A glamorous, charming, and sexual woman, she refused to forget what it was like to be young. At the drop of a straw hat, she and her friends would pack themselves off to Revere Beach, risking the perils of travel through Boston's Irish and Italian outposts for a few rays. And every summer she'd take the three-hour drive through the WASP enclaves of Cape Cod to stay with gay friends who lived in Provincetown. In one photograph in particular we're standing together, arms crossed, me imitating her. She gazes directly into the camera; her hair is blowing, and she's unconcerned about it. That is not a natural look for a colored woman at the beach. She has no scarf binding the hair or cautious hand trying to subdue it.

But as I look at the photo, I can remember how I felt: the roots of my soft, fuzzy hair were pulled tight, locked into braids meant to keep my naps from showing. My grandmother, with her closer link to the Ioway/Wampanoag ancestors, had "good" hair. I did not.

5 When I was a teenager, before leaving for the church dance, I combed my straightened hairdo all to the left side, where I fluffed the luminous curls around my ear. The right side was pulled taut across my head, held by bobby pins and combs. So when I danced with boys I'd have, on one side at least, a vestige of the cascade of curls I'd left home with.

6 I don't know what came over me, or maybe I do. The Black Panther Party was serving free breakfasts in Oakland and carrying guns in public just like John Wayne. Martin Luther King was dead. Africa was more

than just a punch line for comedians' jokes. I now knew that my adolescent hero, Gilda, was not a complete anomaly—there had been African queens. So when my great-grandmother (and guardian) went away to a convention in 1968, I traveled to Beau Brummel Tonsorial Emporium in Roxbury and had my straightened hair cut off by a handsome brother. Dasal Banks wore a vibrant dashiki and the confidence of a young prince. The moment I saw my new self in the mirror, a frisson of fear and recognition rippled through me. When my great-grandmother came home, she squinted at me through glaucoma-clouded eyes and asked what I'd done to my hair. "Nothing," I said, with all the confidence at the disposal of a nineteen-year-old telling a lie. My great-grandmother "umphed" but said no more. Her eyesight wasn't that bad.

7

The "Angelas" never prearranged meetings, we'd simply find ourselves sitting at the same table in the university cafeteria, or after I graduated in 1971, another group of us drifted together over wine in New York cafés. We told stories of what it felt like to know that some people, occasionally the police, suspected you were Angela Davis. The stories varied from routine to hair-raising.

Tall, unstifled, sandy-toned Afro, crowning fair skin, dark eyebrows, and a slight gap in her teeth. Our hero Angela was a fugitive, wanted by the FBI, suspected of taking part in an attempted prison break by black revolutionaries that had left several people dead. She was Bonnie without Clyde, but with a mission instead. I loved the bond we felt with each other and with her. Though fleeting and ephemeral, it was my first sense of a community of women outside my family. So often the Angelas— two or three young women of color, each looking distinctly different from the other—would find ourselves together, wondering what made white people think we were all Angela Davis. The hair, we concluded. The sight of unrestrained, kinky hair scared them so badly they couldn't see anything else. But we saw each other.

8

On her mantel, my mother keeps a carefully framed collection of family portraits going back to my great-great-grandmother. My photos stop twenty-five years ago, at a college picture. I can never decide if that's because it's a picture from before I stopped straightening my hair or because it's from before she knew I was a lesbian.

9 In September 1976 I went, for my birthday, to the Booth Theatre on Broadway to see Ntozake Shange's choreopoem, *For Colored Girls Who Have Considered Suicide/When the Rainbow Is Enuf.* I sat mesmerized, even though I'd seen the performance a dozen times off-Broadway at the Henry Street Settlement. I'd come this time just for the delirious joy of seeing a full cast of colored women and their natural hair on a Broadway stage. Most of my friends who came had naturals or dreadlocks. And the audience was generously sprinkled with other colored lesbians with various natural hairstyles, smiling and greeting each other in public like I'd never seen before. All of the black stars in the audience (like Diana Ross) had hair so done, it was as if the 1960s had never occurred. And those with men sat as stiffly as their processed hair, trying to reveal nothing of their deepest feelings.

10 My lover Sandy, lighting designer and reggae aficionado, started her dreadlocks after hanging out with the Rastas in New York City's Washington Square Park. Thick and black, her hair locked quickly, soon becoming an amazing and glorious mane. But whenever she left the house, I was frightened. It was 1978, and to some on the street, her uncovered locks would mark her as a lesbian and make her a target for violence.

11 "Madeleine's dreads / are weaved on a loom / of balsam flowers / are planted roots / exposed / a forest in a fog / unfathomable." Alexis De-Veaux performed her poem to the rhythm of the shakere played by percussionist Madeleine Nelson. One Sunday a month during the early 1980s the Flamboyant Ladies Salons blossomed at Alexis and Gwen's apartment in Brooklyn. When I close my eyes, I can still see the sway of Madeleine's enormously long dreadlocks and the rapture on the faces of the women who celebrated our hair, our "roots exposed."

12 Almost without a plan, I started locking my hair in 1981. It began to hold just as I started job hunting, so I went to all my interviews wearing scarves and geles carefully chosen to match my outfits. I tried for an academic look halfway between Nation of Islam and Madison Avenue.

13 When I read over the fiction I've written in the past twenty years, I find many places where women of color are combing each other's hair. In my

novel, the main character, named Gilda, is an escaped slave who re-members the feel of her mother's brush in her hair, and it evokes many other forgotten comforts. And later when she combs others' hair, they are usually laughing and telling stories. That particular activity is a nat-ural focus for me—I write about what interests me. Women. And women together. Hair preparation, even when it's torturous, is the time when women (lesbian or not) are totally involved with each other. They can show care for each other, unadorned and unashamed. Or they can pass on self-hatred.

14 In the most recent picture of my stepmother Henrietta, eighty-three, she sports a halo formed by her pure white natural. She's flanked by my younger stepsister, Catherine, and her fourteen-year-old daughter, Atia, both of whom have pressed their hair into obedience, creating patent leather imitations of hair around their gleaming chestnut faces. How did their mother let them leave the house with their hair like that?

15 Recently I've wondered if the myth of the frightening Medusa with her hair of snakes and deadly gaze is not simply the embodiment of people's fear of colored women's hair.

16 The first time a woman touched my dreadlocks, playfully, sensually, I was startled. All of my life women's hair has been made a symbol and a fetish that obscured whatever our own true feelings might be. I've spent years trying to discard the image that had been grafted onto me by oth-ers. Hair is only a part of it. But my ability to renounce an image that felt false to me and build my own began with others' distaste for how I look and how I love. I let go of a cultural construction represented by high school photographs, glossy magazines, advice columns, and swimming caps. It was not a free fall into a void but an ascent, hand over hand, through the braids, plaits, locks, and naps.

When she touched my locks, I wasn't worried they'd "go back" or some other natural disaster. Like my body, my hair was tough and finally my own. In the almost twenty years since, my locks have been short, long, and in between; they've been (courtesy of Lady Clairol) blond, red, auburn, and are now (courtesy of Mother Nature) salt and pepper. And I haven't cursed rainy weather since 1968.

The pressure created by the unrelieved images of black, silky-haired movie stars, middle-class professionals, and singers in popular media—both white and black—is as seductive today as it was thirty years ago or one hundred and thirty years ago. It seduces women away from themselves, away from each other.

I never thought I'd live to see movie stars and notables like Rosalind Cash, Toni Morrison, Whoopi Goldberg, or Alfre Woodard on public stages wearing naturals and dreadlocks, but I have. Even though throughout black communities the hot combs and chemicals still sizzle, Gilda is no longer alone. Some black women have natural waves, others tight curls, others locks. For them and for me the naps are free, the kitchen is not a place of shame. I followed the image of a young woman down the street because it was more compelling than anything else I was being force-fed. And it turned out to be me.

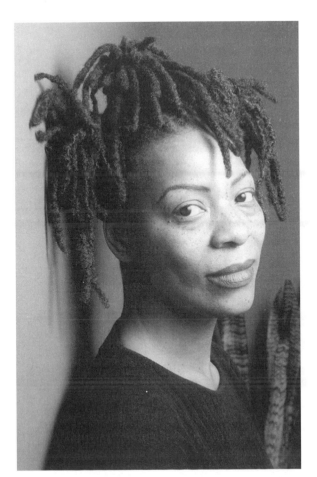

THE CALL
Tamara Jeffries

The voice spoke again. Not so much a voice, really, as an idea that slipped in between the others.

"Cut it," it whispered. "Cut your hair."

Artist Clymenza Hawkins with cascading locks.

CHESTER HIGGINS, JR./
NY TIMES PHOTOS

"Are you kidding?" I quickly dismissed the thought. "I'm not cutting this hair."

I'd been growing my locks for five and a half years, after thirteen years of wearing a short natural. Now the thin, dark ropes reached well past my shoulder blades, striving toward my waist. I had come to love the wild forest they created. It would never have occurred to me to cut it. But that little voice only grew louder.

"Other people cut their locks," it told me.

True.

I thought of my sister, who cut and grew, and then cut and grew her hair so often that I couldn't remember what it looked like from one week to the next. My good girlfriend had taken the scissors to her locks after the birth of her baby; too much work, she'd said. Another sister sheared hers in preparation for a job search, while my cousin lopped off his just because it was time for something new. They all had reasons. I couldn't think of one.

"It's not as if you're Rastafarian. It's not a religion," the voice taunted.

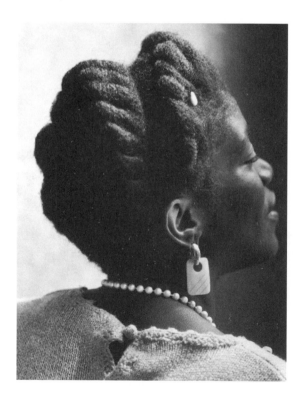

I had always liked locks and enjoyed the freedom from conformity the hairstyle represented. Still, I hadn't started locks with any particular philosophy in mind. I wasn't attached to them for any deeper reason than that I liked the look and the fact that it was compatible with my long-standing commitment to wear my hair natural.

The debate raged on.

"It's just hair. It'll grow back, right?"

New York City, 1989.
A Brooklyn woman.

CHESTER HIGGINS JR.

"It took me too long to grow this hair."

"You didn't grow it," the voice reminded.

No, I did nothing but let it be. The hair grew itself in its own free way.

The voice continued to buzz in my ear. I thought of the Bible's Samson and of those like him who believe that hair has spiritual power that connects you with the universe, with your dreams, with God. "When you cut your hair, Baby-girl," an elder once told me, "you cut your dreams." So of course, the answer was clear: I should keep my hair.

Then I watched Demi Moore in the movie *G.I. Jane,* about the first woman to become a Navy SEAL, shaving away the tresses that got in the way of her goal. My sister, watching beside me, said to the screen, "Go 'head, girl. Feel free, don't you?" which reminded me of the freedom of not having hair in the way, taking up time, needing to be tended. One less thing to think about.

So why did I feel so attached to something as simple and replaceable as hair? I can only say that after five years with the locks, they had become entangled with my identity. They said things about me so I didn't have to. For instance, no matter how conservative I might appear in my pinstripes and pumps, the hair told another tale. To some, it made me unusual, a mystery. It camouflaged my shyness, announcing that I was bold and brave and hip—all things that I, too often, am not.

My choice exempted me from overtly racist employers or men with cultural hangups. If they wanted "straight"—hair or mindset—they'd pass me by. And the locks gained me automatic membership into one or both of two exclusive cultural clubs—the artsy and the Afrocentric. No matter where I went, I could exchange a knowing nod of appreciation and comradeship with someone else wearing locks. I've made lasting friendships initiated by the acknowledgment of that one thing in common. And on the street, I got "Peace, Sista" from brothers who might otherwise have approached with "Hey, slim."

As my hair grew, I enjoyed it billowing behind me in spring storms and winter gusts. When it got long enough, I pulled it into a ponytail or piled it up on my head or braided it, then unbraided so it crinkled. It was beautiful, I thought. My locks became my vanity. I had no need for elaborate jewelry. Makeup was optional. My hair adorned me.

I thought it made me prettier, sexier. And part of it, I had to admit, had to do with ingrained images of voluptuous beauties tossing back manes of hair. The length of my locks saved them even from the "disgrace" of nappiness. Sad as it is, we black girls dreamed of having long hair as we buttoned sweaters on our heads and clipped clothespins to the ends of our pigtails. Lord, we prayed as children (and adults?), let it be long.

The voice, emanating from some hidden part of me, wanted me to give all that up? Speak for myself? Abandon my one, lone vanity? How could I?

One evening, as I sat down to meditate, the voice came to me more soothingly than before. At last, I could no longer resist it. I lit candles and incense, turned on a stream of soft music, and pulled out my grandmother's mirror. Cross-legged on the floor, I began to snip away, without looking. One lock, then another, until each one joined her sisters in a pile on the floor before me.

I made each snip a symbol of commitment. Each strand shorn fell, not on a whim, but in response to a higher urging. Because whose voice was this but that of Spirit? It was testing me, making me go within to ask difficult questions and to examine uneasy answers. It was asking me to grow. The hair piling up on the floor proved that I was willing.

Soon the last dark lock slipped from my hand. I lay down the scissors and reached up to feel the shagginess of what was left. I smiled. The soft hair caressed my fingers. When I felt brave enough to look, I found my face unchanged and the Afro pleasingly familiar. I recognized the young woman in the mirror from high school, and college and my first job. This was a self I knew.

But when I gathered up the shorn locks and held their weight in my hands, salt water dropped from me to them, soaking in, disappearing. The tears had come without warning. As I stroked the dark mass, still warm from the nervous heat of my scalp, I felt as if I'd lost a loved one. Was this just hair in the candlelight shimmering with magnetic energy? It was more than tangled fibers; it was a separate entity, a living thing unto itself. These locks grew out of me, but they weren't a part of me, like my arm, my breast, my ear. No, they were like a child—someone who is of you, but not you. A part of me with a life of its own.

After I'd stood under the hot pulse of the shower washing what was left of my hair, I climbed into bed, exhausted but sleepless. In the dark I lay open-eyed. My head felt cold and naked, with a little spiky itch. But mostly I felt lonely.

Lonely?

I questioned the feeling; loneliness didn't seem appropriate, but there it was. A void that I hadn't felt before opened up within me. The bed that I'd slept in three thousand nights before somehow seemed too big. I was palpably aware of the five states that separated me and my best friend, the weeks since I'd last talked to my mother, the long miles between me and my man. I felt the weight of each day in the years that I'd lived alone, self-sufficient, self-supporting, independent. But alone. I missed my hair, yet felt foolish at the notion. I cried myself to sleep.

It was several days before I could leave my house without feeling naked and anxious and out of sorts. I didn't want anyone I knew to see me. What could they say? Any opinion would nick me too close. The move I'd made was so personal and still too raw.

Outside in the frigid February air, I missed the feeling of my hair in the wind, the warmth of it. I had taken for granted its smell—a wooly fragrance mixed with the undertones of my favorite incense and amber body oil. I longed for my lost forest.

As I traveled through the city, I smiled a knowing greeting to my sisters and brothers with locks, but their return smile seemed less warm. I wasn't a member of the club anymore. I was just another sister on the street. But then again, perhaps there is no club—no affinity beyond the appreciation for kinky, wild hair. Having locks doesn't make one an artist or even particularly Afrocentric. It doesn't make you automatically anything. Were these people with locks like me wearing some kind of easy costume—a soft, nappy armor that says one thing to camouflage or act as a crutch for something else?

Locks, I came to understand, did not define my character. The symbolism of them—the freedom I'd claimed when I made the commitment to grow them against all convention, and the pride in heritage it portrayed—I still owned those things. With or without the extra hair, those qualities grew in my spirit forever.

After a while, I'd catch my reflection in a mirror and wink at the small head, sleek as a bird's. I looked sharp, kinetic, ready, fierce. So now the question remains, will I stick with my dark, close-cropped fuzz? Let it lock again? Grow it into an amazing globe of a 'fro? Braid it, twist it, wrap it—what? I'll just have to see. Right now, I am waiting for The Call.

DON'T NOBODY LAUGH AT HER HAIR

In *Vibration Cooking*, Verta Mae Grosvenor recalls her mother's stories about her sister Rose and their South Carolina childhood. One story is about how Aunt Rose would throw tantrums when she got her hair combed. "This one

Sunday morning Grandmama Sula was combing it for church and she started going through her act. Falling out, calling on the Lord and all; so Grandmamma sent my mother across the swamp to borrow the scissors from cousin Sas P. Ritter. They cut it all off, then got in the horse and buggy and went to Sunday school where everyone laughed at Aunt Rose who promptly cussed them out there and then."

CLEAN BREAK
Jill Nelson

It was not until I was twelve or thirteen, moving into young womanhood with a nascent desire for sexual and physical identity and value, that I was forced to face up to my own invisibility as a black girl. I began to realize that, more often than not, my physical being—brown body, heavy thighs, uncontrollable hair—wasn't seen.

As a child I read "Cinderella," "Sleeping Beauty," "Snow White and the Seven Dwarfs," and "Rapunzel," in which the heroines are always white, always get the prince, live happily ever after, and always, always have long hair. In fact, if Rapunzel hadn't had that long straight hair to let down, the prince wouldn't have had anything to climb up to her tower on, would never have got-

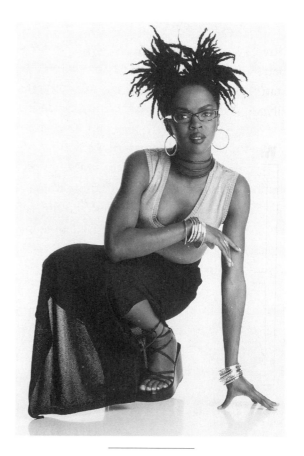

Lauryn Hill spiked.

ANTHONY BARBOZA

ten to her. If I thought as a child these were just fairy tales and not reflections of reality, when I read "The Gift of the Magi" in junior high school English—where the man sells his prized watch to buy a comb for his wife's long, glorious hair, and she simultaneously cuts off her hair, the ultimate sacrifice for love, and sells it to buy him a watch chain—I learned that the importance of long, straight hair was not limited to stories. By adolescence, I knew that it was a point of entry, an attribute that women need to be considered attractive in this culture. As a black girl I learned early on that thick, kinky hair is without value, since rarely are even white women, the embodiment of beauty in a racist culture, with short hair presented as desirable. Hair, and lots of it, is required both for beauty and visibility. It is the beginning of what for most women is a lifelong obsession.

My brother Stanley and I sit on the stoop of the building we live in on 148th Street, before my father's financial success enables us to move downtown, to a better neighborhood, away from black people, which in American culture is up in status. We are hunched over, tightening our roller skates with one of those fat, silver skate keys we used back in the days before Rollerblades. I am nine; my

100 % Humidity
Barbara Brandon
© *1997 Barbara Brandon*

UNIVERSAL PRESS SYNDICATE

brother is ten. He is chocolate-colored, round-faced, with thick kinky hair cut close to the scalp in the style of the day for little black boys, teasingly called a "baldy bean." I am caramel-colored. Except for the difference in our complexions and the texture of our hair, we could pass for twins. My hair is parted in the center and hangs in two braids to the middle of my back. Its texture, closer to the straightness of white people's hair than to the tightly curled hair of black folks, is what black people too often call "good" or "pretty" hair. I learn this from adults, friends of my parents who come to visit and, meeting me, stroke my hair reverentially, an accident of birth or consequence of plantation rape that sets me apart from my sister and two brothers. Even as I enjoy being fawned over, I am made uncomfortable.

Two women walk past, glance our way. They are probably in their early twenties. "Ohhh, look at those long braids," one of the women says.

"Yeah. That girl gotta head of hair."

"She got that pretty hair, too," the woman says. She stops and stands looking down at my brother and me. "Can I touch it?"

I look up at her and for a moment do not know what to say. I want to ask why and then refuse, but I am afraid to, not only because I have been taught to respect adults. I am afraid that to deny this woman's small request will set me apart, make her angry, make her think that I am high siddity, fancy myself better than she.

"Can I touch it, baby?" Her voice is friendly, pleading, demanding, all at once. I nod.

She places both hands on my hairline, her fingertips in the part. She slowly, slowly, runs her hands across the crown, down to where the braids begin. Her fingers wrap my braids within tight fists and continue past the rubber bands, an inch farther to the ends. Her fists hold only air. As long as I live, I will never forget the sensations evoked as this grown-up stranger caressed my hair. I feel simultaneously flattered and embarrassed, complimented and angry, all-powerful and profoundly powerless. "Thank you, baby," she says, and continues up the hill. Unsure what she is thanking me for, I am unable to say, "You're welcome." I don't say anything. Instead, I bend my head down to the task at hand, furiously twisting my skate key. One of my braids falls over my shoulder, swings in front of me. Angrily, I flip it aside. Already finished, Stanley stands up, skates off, disappears around the corner. I hurry to catch up with him.

By the time I am fifteen, in 1967, we no longer live in Harlem, nor do I wear two braids. Four years earlier, when I was eleven, my father's successful dental practice allows him to move us from Harlem to the Upper West Side, to a building in which we are the only black family. My hair is shoulder-length now, and I try to wear it in a flip straight to the collarbone and then ends turned up, kind of like the rich and beautiful Veronica Lodge in the *Archie* comics, although this is not easy. I want to be the Breck Girl from the television and magazine ads, every strand of shining hair always in place. It doesn't work. My hair inevitably balloons.

Most women, white and black, are not comforted by the dominant myths of beauty. The difference for black women is that we do not feel simply ugly, but totally outside, irrelevant, invisible. The significant and continuing success of *Essence* is due in large part to the visibility it gives to black women, in all our diversity of color, hair, and body. Almost three decades after its debut in 1970, *Essence* remains the only magazine that consistently recognizes and embraces the true range of black beauty. In the pages of *Essence*, our beauty is not dependent on our degree of whiteness or the subtle and overt racist and sexist fantasies of male photographers and art directors of black women as exotic, animalistic, overly sexualized objects of domination, degradation, and desire. In these pages, black women's beauty is normal, not aberrant. As a black woman, I have been trying to figure out what is beautiful, and functional, and comfortable for me and my sisters for most of my life.

Over the last ten years I've been having my hair cut shorter and shorter. In the late summer of 1996, when I am forty-four, I have my hair shaved to the scalp with an electric razor. When I leave, my head is covered with a faint memory of brown and silver peach fuzz; I am as close to bald as I can get without lathering up and using a straight razor. I do this because I am tired of everything about hair—having it, combing it, thinking about it, plain feeling it. So, to test my theory that for me hair has finally become obsolete, I got rid of it. I want to see how people react to me, and how I react to myself, hairless. After the first few days, when I wake up startled by my own reflection in the mirror, I come to love it. I like the way it looks, the way it feels bristly when I run my hand over it from any direction, the fact that after four decades I have achieved hair that requires no maintenance.

The response of others is profound. Most black men's eyes skip over me rapidly, distastefully, as if they do not care to see someone who looks like me. I catch pure disdain in the eyes of several. A few stare, look intrigued, and rap to me, although most of these are young enough to be my children. Black women in general—with the exception of the few who are also either bald or wearing short naturals or dreadlocks, who give me a solidarity smile or compliment me—look at me as if I am totally unattractive, insane, and vaguely threatening. It is as if in deciding to be bald I am challenging our collective obsession with hair. Maybe I am. White people, women and men, look surprised and stare at me as I go by. Many people, across race, particularly women, give me a sympathetic smile, assuming, perhaps, that I am a cancer patient undergoing chemotherapy. Whatever a specific individual's response, the most interesting thing about being bald is that I am no longer invisible. Like it or not, everyone sees me. It is a wonderful sensation. Maybe a giant step in black women gaining visibility would be if we all shaved our heads. We would be both immediately visible and connected.

Barring such drastic action, a possible first step would be in acknowledging the commonality of our experiences as black girls and women in a hostile and alien culture. Sometimes that affirmation comes from simply making eye contact. Or talking to girls about self-image. Or teaching young women how to look at popular culture critically. Or telling another woman that she looks nice. That is sisterhood.

Several days after I cut my hair, I walk to the subway station. The woman rapidly climbing the steps ahead of me has dark brown skin, a slim frame. I cannot see how old she is. A teenage girl walks slightly behind her. One of the girl's hands casu-

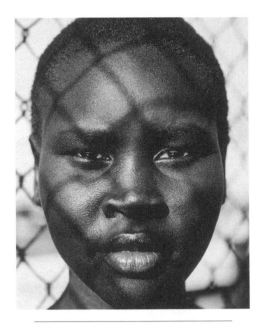

International supermodel Alek Wek makes it with short hair and full features.

CORBIS

▪ 1959 ▪

Lorraine Hansberry's original script for the Broadway production of *A Raisin in the Sun* called for the daughter, "Berneatha" (played by Diana Sands), to wear her hair natural. Just before the play opened, Sands "went natural" at a barbershop, but the style did not work, said Robert Nimiroff, Hansberry's husband. The graceful, tapered, short, feminine au naturel look was not to be had from a quick trip to We Cut Heads in the 'hood barber shop.

ally touches the woman's dreadlocks as she talks. As I close the distance between us, I hear the girl say, "Really Mom, you could go to the hairdresser and they could twist them up right, fix up your locks, they'd look nice. People would notice you, people would be looking from across the street."

The woman turns slightly to look back at her daughter. She is smiling, "Forget it. This ain't no hairstyle," she says as I pull alongside her. She is probably in her early thirties. I reach out my hand, and we slap five, briefly clasp hands, laugh. It is a moment of unspoken understanding, communion, knowing that hair, and so much of what we thought mattered to the business of our being women, doesn't matter at all, or certainly not enough for her to go to a beauty salon and have her low-maintenance dreadlocks styled. It is obsolete. That there is too much work to be done, and that she with her non-salon selected locks and me with my damn near bald head, and all the other sisters struggling for loving self-definition, are bad as we wanna be. At the bottom of the steps her daughter peels off, heading downtown. We climb the last flight of steps in tandem, going in the same direction.

OH, SNAP!

Yo mama hair so short she roll it up with rice.

MY BOLD BLACK STATEMENT
Susan L. Taylor

In the summer of 1970, a sister who was visiting Kenya sent me a postcard with a photograph of an exquisite East African woman with her head shaved.

The image was powerful and captivating. And I learned that the beautifying ritual of shaving their heads had been practiced by Masai women for eons.

I had never seen an image more stunning, more beautiful than the one of that radiant young woman wearing a colorful beaded collar and earrings. But it was more than just her striking physical appearance that called me. She seemed to possess great confidence, an inner connectedness, pure joy. I taped the postcard to my mirror.

I've always worn my hair in ways that are distinctive. And this was 1970, the height of the Black Power Movement, when how you wore your hair was a political statement, and my Harlem sisters and brothers were in serious competition for the fullest, meanest 'fro. I wasn't a competitor in the Afro Wars because my hair is tight and fine, but I decided to make my bold black statement in another way.

Inspired by the image of the Masai woman, I decided to shave my head, leaving only the tiniest fuzz. I loved the freedom of the look, the ease of it all and sitting in the barbershop filled with all those beautiful brothers and getting in and out of there in ten minutes flat. Cutting my hair off was a bodacious move for me. Because I have a high forehead, it seemed hairdressers had tried to give me bangs all of my life. But with no hair, no bangs to hide my naked forehead, no wisps even to veil or frame it, I made peace with it and began, for the first time, to accept and prize my prominent forehead as a unique gift that makes me—and this is true for each of us—a divine original. To this day I've never worn bangs again.

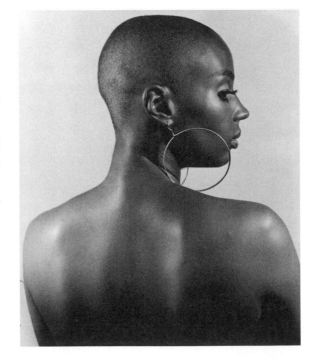

Susan L. Taylor, ca. 1970.

PHOTO KEN RAMSAY

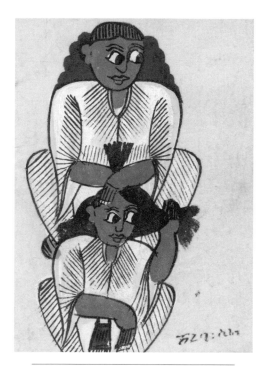

Ethiopian mothers braid their daughters' hair
into a wide array of picturesque styles.

COLLECTION PAMELA JOHNSON

NAPPY BY NATURE

"Now we walk
heads high
naps full of pride
with not a backward glance
at some of the beauty which
used to be."

—from *Hair Raising: Beauty, Culture, and African American Women,*
Noliwe M. Rooks

• 1997 •

According to God, who related it to Carolivia Herron, "One nap of [a black girl's] hair is the only perfect circle in nature."

—from *Nappy Hair,*
Carolivia Herron

POST-TRAUMATIC TRESS SYNDROME

Denise L. Davis, M.D.

She stands motionless and smiling
Brown hair gleaming with carefully applied petroleum products
Her 'do lifelike from camera distance
Dark locks corpse stiff when brushed by lover's fingers
Dry lips stained with color
Thinning her mouth's African fullness
She seems dressed less for success, more for Eternity

There she is, casket-ready, Dr. Miss America
My girlhood illusion sitting cross-legged in the dark
Dreaming of beauty queens and medical school
Fronted by the blue glow of the black-and-white tube
In my imagination, I quaver onto the television set
Waving to crowd, European palm and African fingers
Lifted to greet stricken admirers
My perimenopausal face cosmetized and faintly lined
Will I be able to cry real tears
With rhinestone tiara balanced dangerously
On lye-straightened locks and assimilated brain?
Or will my ducts excrete plastic
Neurotic liquid hardening when it meets air
Falling to the floor like children's pop beads

I wrote this poem, "Dr. Miss America," long after my dreams of glittering tiaras had faded, and my dream of becoming a physician had been achieved. Oakland, California, is my home, a holy and wholly integrated city where kind people sustain me with their compliments about my looks and my long, bushy hair. Paradoxically, I now have no interest in becoming a beauty queen, but I see beauty when I look in the mirror. Competing for approval holds little sway compared to the life of meaning and satisfaction I live as a doctor. I heard the call to healing, and I am grateful. This wasn't always so.

My sixth-grade year ushered in an era of brassieres, makeup, and hair obsession. I began to look into the mirror with critical eyes. My first boy-girl party at John Pittman Elementary marked a tender entry into sexual awareness, while triggering a growing concern about being an outsider in my own community. There were few black families in Kirkwood, Missouri, in 1969. It seemed as if we were integrated into the surrounding suburban white neighborhood, but my looks set me apart.

"Don't take your braids down at school, the other children won't understand your hair." My mother's advice proved accurate when the white boy that I had a deep crush on exclaimed, "Witch!" when he saw my hair after a swim at the pool.

· 1998 ·

Oprah Winfrey explains how she got over her anxieties about her hair "going back" in the cover story of the October *Vogue*. Winfrey had recently done a show with a woman who had written an article about black women and hair. The writer discussed black women's hair obsessions and anxieties and said that this behavior was inhibiting in a number of ways. Agreeing with the writer, Winfrey recalled that when she was first training for the marathon, she didn't want to run in the rain. When her trainer asked why, she replied, "What's wrong wit' you, white boy? . . . I cannot get my hair wet. I will turn to stone." It rained again on the day of the marathon. Winfrey ran it, trampling her H_2O hangup.

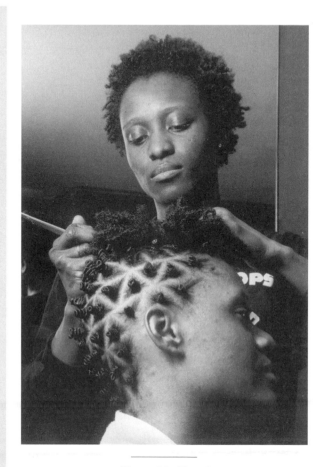

Forget Me Knots!

CHESTER HIGGINS JR.

In *Trauma and Recovery,* Judith Lewis Herman, M.D., writes that the usual response to an emotional or physical blow is to banish the event from consciousness. However, traumatic experience, when denied, can cause later problems. My own desires for different hair and a different life began at age twelve. I hated the way I looked because I didn't have features like the girls in *Teen* magazine; I didn't look like the local homecoming queens; and I was nothing like the girls that my male classmates longed for.

I don't recall a single conversation with Mom or Daddy about our personal encounters with racism. We didn't talk about why my father wore a stocking cap to bed at night, or why my mother was considered to be extraordinarily pretty, in part due to her long, straight hair. Instead, we focused on how a child with beautiful long, kinky hair could have straighter hair with the aid of a Curl Free relaxer, jumbo rollers, and a hair dryer.

Eliciting life histories from patients, says Andrew Weil, M.D., is essential to the practice of good medicine. But we physicians often forget to ask.

If I were my own patient, I might make inquiries into my childhood and ask: How often were the physical features of black people extolled? How often were black women held up as a model for the beauty of the human body? Having one's antennae up for rejection is an expected response and adaptation to hurtful experience. "Flashbacks" are also a normal response to stress.

Today as a doctor of internal medicine, I've come to understand that I can provide the most compassionate and effective care when I know the source of the ailment. And behavior that may seem "crazy" usually has a layer of logic if you review the situation in which the conduct takes place—past and present. In a world where Caucasian notions of beauty dominate, it makes sense that women and men try to change their locks to approximate the dominant notion of beauty, even if the regimen includes hot combs and lye. Hair care is a body and soul issue.

The wounds of racism are evident at cosmetic counters, in mass media, as well as in the physician's office. bell hooks recounts how frequently black women with natural hairstyles have heard, "You could be fine if you did something with that hair." This seemingly minor trauma has resulted in scores of women seeing themselves as unattractive. For example, a Jewish woman in my community asks her husband before she rushes to the office, "Is my hair too big?" meaning too kinky. She reports being extremely sensitive, "hyperaroused," to the looks and comments of others, regarding her hair.

I have often walked into a room full of strangers, wondering if I would be rejected because of my hair, even when the reality is that I'm usually warmly welcomed in professional and social situations. I am, at some level, still the girl in the rain with my hair shrinking into tighter curls as schoolmates stare at me. Often we forget to remember.

When I began to ask my patients how they feel about their hair, and in what ways their hair-care regimen affects their life, they began to look back. A woman in her twenties told me that she will not exercise vigorously, because it disturbs her straightened hairdo. She learned early that straightened hair is beautiful, and that natural hairstyles are less attractive. Who doesn't want to be counted among the beautiful?

Another patient, an elderly woman with arthritis, declines my suggestion for pool exercise because she doesn't want to risk getting her hair wet. These decisions are not based on ignorance, they are an adaptation to the world in which we live, and they are choices that have potentially negative health consequences.

I've seen women with bald spots from the traction of the rollers they use to achieve that smooth, sophisticated look. I've made referrals to dermatologists for my African-American women patients who are losing their hair due to relaxer treatments. And I've received dermatology consult letters recommending that women stop using all the chemicals and heat in order to arrest the process of alopecia—a loss of hair.

How can we begin to heal?

Herman writes that the first step in recovery from traumatic events is establishing personal and collective safety. Living in a safe environment may sound simple, but it is not easy. On the most basic level, in order to heal, men and women need freedom from threats to the body. Physical safety includes the liberty to move about without the threat of assault. In many neighborhoods and places of work, this kind of safety is not yet a reality. And though the threat or the reality of assault may not have a direct connection to appearance (or hairstyle), every wound impacts on the psyche. The thinking goes somewhat like this: "If I am mistreated, or in constant danger of being mistreated, and few come to my defense, something must be wrong with me." This thinking is often subtle or wholly unconscious; but it messes with our heads in more ways than one.

Abraham Maslow's hierarchy-of-needs theory is applicable to recovery from post-traumatic (s)tress syndrome. In Maslow's system, women and men become "self-actualized" only after the most basic survival needs have been met. In order to love and affrim our God-given attributes, we need to create environments that are relatively free of violence, where we have adequate health care, where we are not physically exploited.

Our emotions must also be held sacred. It's not just okay to cry, it's normal and necessary. Grieving is a normal response to loss and is a process that leads to growth. Perhaps we need a moment of silence for every time the light went out in a black girl's eyes because society convinced her that beauty was beyond her grasp. After that we can weep and moan, and begin to take notice of the new life that is being born.

Ideas ought to be held safe, too. It is our right and our duty to think critically about our world and about how many of our ideas about our looks come from internalized racism. We need to analyze the origins of our belief systems about male and female beauty, and stop idolizing an ideal of attractiveness that doesn't even serve the majority!

There is no shame in owning up to the real effects of traumatic experience. Understanding the literature about the consequences of trauma on human beings can help us recover. We are all vulnerable to the effects of trauma, whether we are victims of ill treatment or witnesses to it.

We need the love and support of each other regarding hairstyles, natural or processed. Smiling at another African-American woman is an act of defiance, putting the lie to the myth that we can't appreciate each other. I would go so far as to say that a compliment given to a woman of African descent is a healing and subversive act. The dominant Caucasian paradigm of beauty is overthrown. Paradoxically, I do not believe that our compliments need be politically correct. My own experience is that receiving positive comments about how I look, whether my hair is straight or nappy, allows me to believe that I am attractive in many different situations.

I now live far from where I was a sixth-grader, in a place where I feel deeply appreciated for who I am, what I do, and how I look. When my youngest stepdaughter, who is white, told me that she loves how I look with my natural hair texture, and with little or no makeup, I began to feel freer to go public with my more "organic" look.

After a person feels safe, she can begin the process of remembering the specific details of past harms. This aids in healing. But recalling the truth requires courage as well as social and spiritual support. My patients continue to depend on hairstyles that harm their hair and their scalp because we continue to bear up under the unequal and unfair treatment that began when we were Africans torn from our land and enslaved by Europeans. Sorely missing in our communities are groups where the painful and personal wounds of racism can be remembered in the presence of loving witnesses. Too often experiences of racism are private wounds that twist our public behavior. We need to have sessions where we tell the story of our s/tresses—the truth about our experience and our hair.

After we find safety, after we remember the source of our injuries, we can then reconnect to the beauty of our bodies, the strength in our souls, and the gift of our newfound crowning glory.

FROM SEA TO SHINE

I am my mother's daughter
who puts me in the water
to see if I could swim.
My hair went back to Africa.

—Harryette Mullen

IN SICKNESS AND IN HEALTH
Frankie Alexander

"All that pretty hair," moaned Margaree, my hairdresser, as I sat there waiting for it to fall all over me and onto the floor.

"Yeah," I said halfheartedly, but the hair was an unwelcome weight at that moment. Its removal seemed as critical as pulling an aching tooth. Almost two weeks had passed since I was released from the hospital, and my hair was driving me crazy! It stayed under control when I was in the hospital, or maybe being hooked up to machines like a car battery and dealing with all the anxiety made me oblivious to my hair. But now that I was home, I was eager to cut it off. I had lost ten pounds, and my face looked narrow. But once the hair was gone, my face looked smaller still. I felt so vulnerable.

That night, though, when I settled into my bed, I felt a surge of joy: My pillow felt delicious against my scalp. The sensation was so foreign that it seemed I had never known it, even though I wore my hair short in college. As I lay there, I remembered all the frustrations I'd been through with my hair in the past. For all the confusion and uncertainty a cancer diagnosis had brought into my life, at that moment, my hair and I were at peace.

The turmoil had begun after years of perfect checkups and menstrual cycles that I could have set my clock by. I felt the pains in my pelvic area. They were sharp and sudden, but they didn't last long. I kept telling myself to make an appointment to see my gynecologist, and after almost two months I finally did.

"I noticed you jumped when I felt your left ovary," my gynecologist told me after I'd dressed. "I felt a cyst on that ovary. It's small—about the size of a golf ball."

Those words ushered in a major change in my life. An ultrasound showed that the golf ball was not a cyst, nor would it dissolve as easily as it had erupted. Instead it showed bilateral tumors that were growing on my ovaries. I couldn't believe it. I always prided myself on watching my diet and exercising—doing all the "right" things. It was hard to believe I might have cancer. But this was a real possibility.

The ultrasound, coupled with an elevated CA125, a test that measures hormone levels in the blood, convinced my doctor that surgery was needed immediately. He said they would go in, remove the tumors, and do a frozen-section analysis to check for cancerous cells. If there was no cancer, the surgery would be finished. If the tumors were cancerous, more extensive surgery would be needed. I was forty-one and had never been hospitalized. I was scared.

The frozen section of tissue confirmed the cancer, and I had to have a complete hysterectomy. Still, my doctor said I was not out of the woods yet. We had to wait for the full pathology report. For four days, I lay in the hospital bed wondering whether I'd be told that I only had a few months to live. Finally, the report arrived.

When my doctor came into the room, I saw a slight smile on his face. "Six cycles of chemotherapy," he announced. It was a prophylactic measure, he explained. I was grateful that the cancer had not spread to my lymph nodes and that the surgery was successful, but the prospect of having chemotherapy made me feel hopeless. I worried about this next new unknown. Would I become bald? Would I ever feel normal again?

Before I started the chemo, one of the nurses told me that I would probably want to get my hair cut. She said she couldn't predict whether I would lose my hair, but I should cut it gradually, and then it wouldn't be as big a shock if the chemo took it out.

I was in need of a perm before I had the surgery, so by this time I had a good two or three inches of untreated hair. The incision from the surgery was painful, and the thought of having my arms up for any major length of time to fiddle with my hair was not at all appealing. So I decided not to do the gradual hair-cutting, but to go straight for the close-cut natural. I was prepared to meet chemotherapy head-on.

I've been cancer free and hair free for more than five years now. I suppose there's always the fear of recurrence in the back of the mind of anyone who's had cancer. In my own experience, I've tried to eliminate as much toxicity from my environment and body as I can—that's included staying away from hair relaxers. So, I've basically worn the same style, a close 'fro, for these five years, which can be daunting. While doing volunteer work for Habitat for Humanity, for instance, I heard some sorority sisters from North Carolina Central University lamenting their hair woes. I went on about my work, unloading sacks of sandwiches from my car for the crew's lunch, but I became aware, by their looks, that they were commenting (perhaps unflatteringly) on my hair. Rather than be offended, I smiled, glad to be alive, hair or no hair.

HOLY HAIR
Numbers 6:5

All the days of the vow of his separation there shall be no razor come upon his head until the days be fulfilled in which he separateth himself unto the Lord, he shall be holy and shall the locks of the hair of his head grow.

OPPRESSED HAIR PUTS A CEILING ON THE BRAIN
Alice Walker

This was a talk I gave on Founders' Day, April 11, 1987, at Spelman College in Atlanta:

As some of you no doubt know, I myself was a student here once, many moons ago. I used to sit in these very seats (sometimes still in pajamas, underneath my coat) and gaze up at the light streaming through these very windows. I listened to dozens of encouraging speakers, and sang and listened to wonderful music. I believe I sensed I would one day return, to be on this side of the podium. I think that, all those years ago, when I was a student here and still in my teens, I was thinking about what I would say to you now.

It may surprise you that I do not intend (until the question-and-answer period perhaps) to speak of war and peace, the economy, racism or sexism, or the triumphs and tribulations of black people or of women. Or even about movies. Though the discerning ear may hear my concern for some of these things in what I am about to say, I am going to talk about an issue even closer to home. I am going to talk to you about hair. Don't give a thought to the state of yours at the moment. Don't be at all alarmed. This is not an appraisal. I simply want to share with you some of my own experiences with our friend hair, and at the most hope to entertain and amuse you.

For a long time, from babyhood through young adulthood mainly, we grow, physically and spiritually (including the intellectual with the spiritual), without being deeply aware of it. In fact, some periods of our growth are so confusing that we don't even recognize that growth is happening. We may feel hostile or angry or weepy and hysterical, or we may feel depressed. It would never occur to us, unless we stumbled on a book or person who explained to us, that we were in fact in the process of change, of actually becoming larger, spiritually, than we were before. Whenever we grow, we tend to feel it, as a young seed must feel the weight and inertia of the earth as it seeks to break out of its shell on its way to becoming a plant. Often the feeling is anything but pleasant. But what is most unpleasant is the not knowing what is happening. I remember the waves of anxiety that used to engulf me at different periods in my life, always manifesting itself in physical disorders (sleeplessness, for instance), and how frightened I was because I did not understand how this was possible.

With age and experience, you will be happy to know, growth becomes a conscious, recognized process—still somewhat frightening, but at least understood for what it is. Those long periods when something inside ourselves seems to be waiting, holding its breath, unsure about what the next step should be, eventually become the periods we wait for, for it is in those periods that we realize that we are being prepared for the next phase of our life and that, in all probability, a new level of the personality is about to be revealed.

A few years ago, I experienced one such long period of restlessness disguised as stillness. That is to say, I pretty much withdrew from the larger world in favor

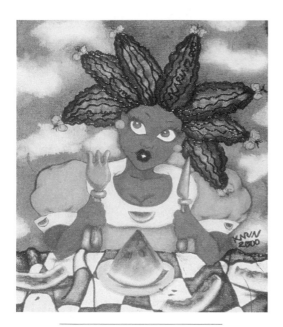

Next Helping of Love, Please.
Acrylic, 2000.

KARIN TURNER

of the peace of my personal, smaller one. I unplugged myself from television and newspapers (a great relief!), from the more disturbing member of my extended family, and from most of my friends. I seemed to have reached a ceiling in my brain. And under this ceiling my mind was very restless, although all else about me was calm.

As one does in these periods of introspection, I counted the beads of my progress in this world. In my relationship to my family and the ancestors, I felt I had behaved respectfully (not all of them would agree, no doubt); in my work I felt I had done, to the best of my ability, all that was required of me; in my relationship to the persons with whom I daily shared my life, I had acted with all the love I could possibly locate within myself. I was also at least beginning to acknowledge my huge responsibility to the earth and my adoration of the universe. What else, then, was required? Why was it that, when I meditated and sought the escape hatch at the top of my brain, which, at an earlier stage of growth, I had been fortunate enough to find, I now encountered a ceiling, as if the route to merge with the infinite I had become used to was plastered over?

One day, after I had asked this question earnestly for half a year, it occurred to me that in my physical self there remained one last barrier to my spiritual liberation, at least in the present phase: my hair.

Not my friend hair itself, for I quickly understood that it was innocent. It was the way I related to it that was the problem. I was always thinking about it. So much so that if my spirit had been a balloon eager to soar away and merge with the infinite, my hair would be the rock that anchored it to Earth. I realized that there was no hope of continuing my spiritual development, no hope of future growth of my soul, no hope of really being able to stare at the universe and forget myself entirely in the staring (one of the purest joys!) if I still remained chained to thoughts about my hair. I suddenly understood why nuns and monks shaved their heads!

I looked at myself in the mirror, and I laughed with happiness! I had broken through the seed skin, and was on my way upward through the earth.

Now I began to experiment. For several months I wore long braids (a fashion among black women at the time) made from the hair of Korean women. I loved this. It fulfilled my fantasy of having very long hair, and it gave my short, mildly processed (oppressed) hair a chance to grow out. The young woman who braided my hair was someone I grew to love—a struggling young mother, she and her daughter would arrive at my house at seven in the evening, and we would talk, listen to music and eat pizza or burritos while she worked, until one or two o'clock in the morning. I loved the craft involved in the designs she created on my head. (Basket making! a friend once cried on feeling the intricate weaving atop my head.) I loved sitting between her knees the way I used to sit between my mother's and sister's knees while they braided my hair when I was a child. I loved the fact that my own hair grew out and grew healthy under the "extensions," as the lengths of hair were called. I loved paying a young sister for work that was truly original and very much a part of the black hairstyling tradition. I loved the fact that I did not have to deal with my hair except once every two or three months (for the first time in my life I could wash it every day if I wanted to and not have to do anything further.). Still, eventually the braids would have to be taken down (a four-to-seven-hour job) and redone (another seven to eight hours); nor did I ever quite forget the Korean women, who, according to my young hairdresser, grew their hair expressly to be sold. Naturally this information caused me to wonder (and, yes, worry) about all other areas of their lives.

When my hair was four inches long, I dispensed with the hair of my Korean sisters and braided my own. It was only then that I became reacquainted with its natural character. I found it to be springy, soft, almost sensually responsive to moisture. As the little braids spun off in all directions but the ones I tried to encourage them to go, I discovered my hair's willfulness, so like my own! I saw that my friend hair, given its own life, had a sense of humor. I discovered I liked it.

Again I stood in front of the mirror and looked at myself and laughed. My hair was one of those odd, amazing, unbelievable, stop-you-in-your-tracks creations—not unlike a zebra's stripes, an armadillo's ears, or the feet of the electric-blue-footed boobie—that the universe makes for no reason other than to express its own limitless imagination. I realized I had never been given the opportunity to appreciate hair for its true self. That it did, in fact, have one. I remember years of enduring hairdressers—from my mother onward—doing missionary work on my hair. They dominated, suppressed, controlled. Now more or less free, it stood this way and that. I would call up my friends around the country to report on its antics. It never thought of lying down. Flatness, the missionary position, did not interest it. It grew. Being short, cropped off near the root, another missionary "solution," did not interest it either. It sought more and more space, more light, more of itself. It loved to be washed, but that was it.

Eventually I knew precisely what hair wanted: it wanted to grow, to be itself, to attract lint, if that was its destiny, but to be left alone by anyone, including me, who did not love it as it was. What do you think happened? (Other than that I was now able, as an added bonus, to comprehend Bob Marley as the mystic his music has always indicated he was.) The ceiling at the top of my brain lifted; once again my mind (and spirit) could get outside myself. I would not be stuck in restless stillness, but would continue to grow. The plant was above ground!

This was the gift of my growth during my fortieth year. This and the realization that as long as there is joy in creation, there will always be new creations to discover, or rediscover, and that a prime place to look is within and about the self. That even death, being part of life, must offer at least one moment of delight.

A GIFT OF LOVE

In Sierra Leone's Mende culture, offering to plait another woman's hair is a way of asking her to become your friend. A beautiful, distinctive style is considered a gift of love, that is, one woman saying to another: "I like you. I appreciate you. I have thought about you enough to imagine a style that will suit and enhance your features. I am not jealous of you. I want you to look beautiful so that you will attract love, admiration, and all the good that these bring. I am willing to stand or bend for several hours, working on your hair, expecting no remuneration. My sacrifice proves that I want only the best for you."

—Sylvia Boone, *Radiance in the Waters: Ideals of Feminine Beauty in Mende Art*

A HAPPY NAPPY HAIR-CARE AFFAIR
Linda Jones

Greetings: I'm having a small gathering of sistas at my house to deal with the oft-heard lament of what to do with our hair. This is primarily for my sistas who can't find a stylist to help them groom their locks. I figure, why can't we just get together and do our own? So there. We will be sitting on my back deck, washing and twisting hair and massaging scalps. Casual, of course. Come relax and commune. This is my happy nappy hair-care affair. (Got a few shine heads and perms comin', but we ain't mad at 'em!)

> **• ALL IN ONE •**
>
> Discovering your own beauty has repercussions far beyond the self. As East Indian philosopher Radhakrishnan says, "These two elements of selfhood, uniqueness (each-ness) and universality (all-ness) grow together until at last the most unique becomes the most universal."

My Happy Nappy Hair-Care Affair was intended to be a simple grassroots grooming session. It was an opportunity for me and my girlfriends to get together on a Sunday afternoon and do our own hair. There were some who thought I was trying to revive an African tradition. A friend who visited Nigeria recently told me that Sunday is a day women get together to do their hair for the week to come. But as much as I embrace some traditions of the motherland, what I had in mind when I decided to have my gathering wasn't that deep. All I wanted to do was to offer a place for my friends who wear African-inspired and natural hairstyles to come and get their hair groomed for free and be among kindred spirits. At my house their heads would not stand out in the crowd. On that one afternoon, they could be assured they would have majority status. They would be the rule, not the exception.

I was hoping that my hair affair would help my friend Ruth, for example, find someone to help tighten up the new growth of dreadlocks in the back of her head where she couldn't reach. I knew my friend Barbara, who wanted to switch her micro-'fro to micro-twists, was in search of someone with the patience and fingers nimble enough to help her make the transition, and I wanted to help my coworker Halimah, who was new to Dallas and had limited funds, meet someone

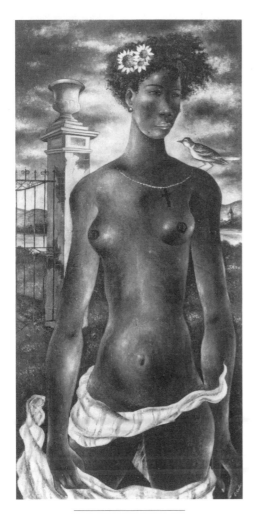

Southern Gate, ca. 1942.

Oil on canvas.

ELDZIER CORTOR

NATIONAL MUSEUM OF AMERICAN

ART, WASHINGTON, D.C./ART

RESOURCE, N.Y.

to help her groom her locks until she could find an affordable loctician.

I also had selfish reasons for sponsoring this event. I wanted to be transported back to my childhood. I missed the moment of bonding when the females in our household got together to do hair. I am not referring to the traumatic Saturday-night rituals when my mother fried our hair in preparation for church on Sunday morning. The sight of her brandishing that hot comb, the hissing sound it made when it came into contact with my grease-laden hair, and the peculiar smell of something burning on my head made me wish I was born bald.

What I missed were the more natural moments, when my mother placed her healing hands directly on my head. I remembered how comforting it was nestling between her strong knees as she oiled and massaged my scalp with her fingers before brushing, combing, and arranging my hair into a simple style of plaits or ponytails. I would lean back, close my eyes, and surrender to her firm but gentle touch. Being the eldest daughter, I often did my younger sisters' hair, and when my mother was too tired to do her own, we would do it for her. Those were the times when we were closest. Having the hair affair would give me an opportunity to re-create such moments at my home, with my extended family of sister friends.

I got the idea one day at work after listening to Halimah's latest lament about being unable to find the right hairstylist. As a temporary solution, I suggested she come to my house, and we could do each other's hair. I told her I knew other women with similar concerns, so we could make it a communal affair. I decided to have it on the third Sunday in May 1998. It was an experiment. I didn't really know what to expect. I never imagined that two years later, I would still be having what the regulars have now dubbed "hair day."

The first gathering was so well received that I was urged to have them on a regular basis. Since my work as a journalist is demanding, I could only commit to having the gatherings every other month. Gradually, others began to sponsor sessions in between.

Hair day has evolved into much more than a grooming session. At these gatherings the women have formed a circle of solidarity and support. We have celebrated our hair through storytelling and poetry readings and endless testimonials about our journey to appreciate ourselves as we really are. Hair day is a time when my sisters come to vent about those who have judged them harshly for their choice to be themselves. On that day they are able to decompress. Our circle is an eclectic mix of Ivy League pedigrees and sisters with no degrees. We have mothers, daughters, women who work, and women in transition. Some are lesbians, others straight. There are artists and writers, teachers and students, computer nerds, probation officers, African dancers, and sisters who drum. We try to keep things simple and positive. Some of the regular "napaholics" are so protective of our circle that they refuse to tell others about it. They fear it will lose its intimacy or be tarnished by negative personalities. Others have been so inspired by the experience that they can't wait to spread the word.

It wasn't long before "hair day" became the catalyst for another project I inadvertently got myself into. While preparing a note to send to the regular members reminding them when my next bimonthly gathering would be, I decided to include a few brief items about natural hair issues I knew about.

I wrote about the white elementary school teacher in New York who drew criticism from black parents for reading *Nappy Hair*—a positive story about just that—to her black and Latino students. I wrote about the first annual dreadlock summit in Texas and about the sister in North Carolina who was repeatedly banned from participating in a sorority debutante ball because the organization didn't feel that her dreadlocks were appropriate for the formal occasion.

Next thing I knew my "note" became a newsletter. I became the dreadlocked "head-itor" of *Nappy News*, and my partner, Yvette Robinson, another wordsmith who sports a low natural, serves as the second "bush-mama-in-charge." Are we having fun yet? Do you really need to ask? The sessions have struck the women in ways I never imagined.

Audra, a twenty-one-year-old graduate from the University of Alabama who came to my July session while in town visiting Halimah, found it to be cathartic. It had been nearly two years since Audra lost her mother to breast cancer, and since she wanted to be strong for her father and brothers, she kept her emotions to herself. One of the women she met at my gathering was Alpha, a breast cancer survivor who was forced to cut her dreadlocks while undergoing treatment. She still wears her hair naturally, in a midsize

> • A PEACHY RECIPE •
> FOR SHINY HAIR
>
> Here's a hair-care recipe from Mother Gwen Swinton, one of our hair-day regulars. She says the minerals in the leaves of a peach make your hair shine and your scalp feel rejuvenated. Mother Swinton got the recipe from her mother, who's 101 years old:
>
> "Boil a pot of peach tree leaves, let it cool, add vinegar then set the mixture aside. Shampoo & rinse your hair. Pour the mixture through the hair & massage in well. Leave it in for two minutes then rinse out."
>
> —*Nappy Hair Care Affair Newsletter*

Afro, and courageously takes her condition, which is now in remission, in stride. Audra overheard Alpha talking about her challenges and was uplifted by her words. She was also befriended by Cathi, who arranged her shoulder-length hair into an attractive style of flat twists and Bantu knots. Since Audra wasn't adept at doing hair, she offered Cathi and others free massages in return. The nurturing she received from the women that day brought back fond memories of her mother and filled her with such emotion that later that evening she was finally able to release the tears she had been holding back for so long.

"I can't describe it in words," she told me about her visit and the feelings it evoked. "The women just made me feel at ease."

My friend Cheri, who wears her hair so short you can see what's on her mind, came to her first hair day in September 1998. "I only attended one session, but I really felt part of the group," she said. "You didn't have to put on a front, and you could have a good time. There was no backbiting, and nobody was tearing anybody down."

My friends who wear perms were even intrigued by the concept of my nappy hair affair. One even got offended when she didn't get an invitation to my first one. "So is my hair not nappy enough?" Renee asked me. For obvious reasons I didn't think she'd be interested, but she knew that I invited another friend who also wears a perm.

"My hair is nappier than hers," she whined. To prove it, Renee proceeded to part her relaxed hair with her fingers to show me her new growth. I couldn't believe I was watching a straight-haired sister trying to outnap another straight-haired sister. I was flattered and amused. Renee wanted so much to come to my nappy hair affair that she tried to produce enough kinks to qualify for admission. I told her that wasn't necessary, and invited her to come anyway. I guess all she wanted was the invitation, because she never showed up.

But many others did. Twenty women with skin kissed by the sun gathered in my backyard on that warm spring Sunday afternoon and transformed it into a garden of dreadlocks, twists, Bantu knots, braids, and Afros in full bloom. The first to arrive found me getting a massage in the shade of my pecan tree, and not about to move. Since I was a bit nervous about hosting my first hair-grooming session, I needed someone to work the kinks out of my body before anyone got to my head. Cynthia, who makes her living as a massage therapist, came early to oblige.

To help my guests get acclimated, I posted a sign in the kitchen:

> *Welcome to My Happy Nappy Hair Care Affair.*
> *Make yourself at home. Find a seat on a chair, on*
> *the floor. Help yourself to whatever you brought*
> *to eat. But don't bother me because I'm getting my*
> *hair "did." You best find someone to do yours . . .*

The message was clear. This was an unstructured, self-serve hair-care affair. Things fell right into place. Those who had visited my home before helped the newcomers get situated. My home is a no-shoe zone, and my guests seemed more than willing to shed their footwear and get on common ground. They deposited their pot-luck dishes in the kitchen, then returned to the backyard, where they gravitated toward my patio deck and briefly exchanged greetings before moving quickly to the topic of hair.

Every conceivable area was covered. They swapped hair-care recipes—like how witch hazel reduces buildup in dreadlocks and how lemon juice keeps them tight. They shared hair taboo and superstitions:

HALIMAH: My grandmother says it's bad luck to have your [cut] hair laying out. You have to bury it.
RUTH: I buried mine once in a rich neighborhood.
BENITA: So are you rich?
RUTH: Not yet.

Adult survivors of the hot comb offered amusing testimonials.

ROSALIND: My aunt's thing was to talk on the phone and pop gum while she was burning my hair. She would say, "Oh, did that burn you?" I'd tell her, "Oh, no, I'm just about to fall out of the chair. But I'm not on fire . . ."

Unflattering names for nappy-headed people were resurrected for review.

BENITA: "Chicken head? I think that's a southern thing. I've heard about that ever since I was a little girl. When you have short hair and it's nappy, you're called a chicken head. It is not a compliment."

Taking a break from massaging the sisters who had kept her busy all afternoon, Cynthia shared her story of what happened when she tried to relax her thick head of hair, which apparently had a mind of its own. She spoke as though she was making a confession and was almost apologetic when she told us what she had done. We struggled not to laugh too hard at her heartfelt but humorous story:

"I had natural hair since '92, until a week ago. . . . It had gotten to the point where I couldn't find anyone to [help me] do it. So last week I got an hour perm and it still didn't take . . . it still didn't take." She pointed to her head to show the result of her failed attempt to get her willful hair to submit. The top was braided in cornrows that met in a fuzzy puff at the top, and the texture of it hovered somewhere between nappy and straight.

Eventually the women got around to what the gathering was all about. They chose partners and got busy grooming hair. A few retreated to the bathroom for a shampoo, but most of them had washed their hair before they came and were eager to get started on a style. They worked to the reggae, merengue, salsa, and jazz that I had loaded in my CD player.

It was a beautiful portrait. Some worked while standing, others sat in stairstep fashion, palm rolling, twisting, or otherwise fussing over the head of the person in front of them. Their arms were extended like branches of a family tree and moving nonstop. Watching them work reminded me of a painting by Boston-based artist Paul Goodnight. The painting, called *Links and Lineage*, depicts a family of black women—from the elderly matriarch to the youngest girl—engaged in the ritual of grooming each other's hair. What was happening on my deck was like seeing Goodnight's painting come to life.

Denise, one of the "token perms" who came, was so moved by what she witnessed in my backyard that afternoon that she called for one of us to take her back to her roots. She asked me for a pair of scissors. "Does anyone know how to cut hair?" she asked. There was no professional hairstylist or barber among us, but that didn't matter to Denise, who insisted that someone cut away all traces of her relaxed hair.

Annette, a willowy visual artist who wears a short natural, took up the scissors and the challenge. The most experience Annette has had in cutting hair was when she cut her own locks and used them in her artwork. She is most known for a series of pieces where she arranged dates of her first menstrual cycle to the most recent, in spiral patterns, incorporating drops from her menstual flow into the work. She calls the series *Drawing Blood*. It was exhibitied at the Whitney Museum in New York. We assured Denise that would not be happening on her head. Denise wasn't worried. "If there was ever a time to do this, it is today."

Denise settled into a patio chair, and Annette handled her head like it was a sculpture. She took her time, and for most of an hour she meticulously snipped and shaped until all that was left when she finished was a short, wooly layer of virgin hair softly framing Denise's face. The complete work of art drew applause from the sisters on the sidelines and a warm hug from Denise, who was ecstatic over her new natural look.

"I feel good," Denise squealed after we convinced her to put the mirror away. "I feel light . . . I feel free." Watching Denise blossom after Annette's shearing—they formed a bond of friendship that still exists today—was for me the most powerful moment of the evening.

Not only did I not have any grand intentions when I decided to have my nappy hair affair, I didn't even think beyond that first one. Yet it evolved into more than I ever thought it would be. That's the beauty of it.

Since hair day is still going on, there really is no ending to my story. Our gatherings have become so popular that brothers have even started complaining about being excluded. One even threatened to picket outside my house during our session. While I'm thinking about having a special day for them when we can teach them how to "bond," then send them off to have their own sessions, I intend to preserve the female sanctity of our circle. And as busy as I am, I don't intend to stop having hair day any time soon. There's too much healing going on.

Ms. Strand Adjourns

The tenderheads gathered back in the auditorium after submitting their essays, poetry, and art work. Halima was resplendent in her turquoise, burgundy and gold gele. Jenyne was rocking the flip. And Nikky's locks had the earthy scents of lavender and rosemary. Each contributor was beautiful in her or his own way. And each was humming with the excitement of discovery. As Ms. Strand strolled to the mike, the room fell silent. They strained to hear her soft voice.

"Tenderheads, I want to thank you for the fine work you've done. I know figuring out our hair is hard, but you did it—masterfully. So, are there any questions?"

Several contributors' hands flew up. Ms. Strand pointed to one near the back. "Yes?"

"Ms. Strand, this whole process has been cathartic. I got so much out of it but what do you tell the average black woman about doing her hair on the average day?"

"Know your own head. Sometimes we turn our heads over to others, and lose touch with them. Your head is not only for public display. Even if you choose to conform, for whatever reason, it's still your personal space. Never forget that. Experiment with who you are and what you want to say—even with your hair. Spend some time with it when nobody's looking. Love it, encourage it."

"Ms. Strand, over here."

"Yes."

"Some people, and I won't mention names, feel that the longer and smoother your hair is, the better it looks, and the better chance you have to get all the prizes."

"And too often that's still true. But that ends up leaving a lot of us out and dividing us. We need to compliment one another, share ideas and find ways to beautify ourselves that keep changing to fit the people we are becoming."

"Ms. Strand, what message should we take to our little girls?"

"We have to be aware of the messages they're getting from us without our even saying anything. Maybe the most innovative thing that we can do is to reach back and get those old African traditions, where hairstyles had names and meanings and mottoes. When we do this, it will no longer be about little girls saying, 'You think you cute because you got long hair.' Every girl could be cute because her hairstyle, whatever its length, would be uniquely suited to her and would speak volumes. The older girls and women in the community could help with this by selecting styles to suit each girl based on her personality, her face and her body type. These styles would be as infinite as imagination and as personal as a signature. And the meanings could be imparted during a special ceremony. A star-burst pattern would have a name like 'Galaxy Dancer,' with a sweet little song to go with it, like 'Galaxy Dancer is so fly because her head is to the sky.'"

The passionate discussion heated the room. Ms. Strand began to perspire, and then she began to shrink. The humidity had gotten to her and she was no longer tall enough to reach the mike. So people came close to hear, and she spoke in her natural voice:

"We've learned a lot here, and I invite y'all to keep thinking on these questions. But don't let them weigh you down."

Ms. Strand sighed, satisfied. Her kinky, curly, wavy, and occasionally straight story, had finally been told.

About the Contributors

Frankie Alexander, an independent writer and jazz vocalist, is an administrator at Duke Medical Center in Durham, North Carolina.

Annabelle Baker is a retired nurse in New York City.

Idara Bassey is an attorney, writer, and mixed-media artist based in the Washington, D.C., area.

Kay Brown, an independent writer who lives in Washington, D.C., is completing a book on the history of the 1960s black arts movement, of which she was a part.

A'Lelia Bundles, author of *Madam C. J. Walker: A Family Legacy* (Scribner, 2001), is a former Washington deputy bureau chief for ABC News.

Lucille Clifton is Distinguished Professor of Humanities at St. Mary's College in Maryland and the author of numerous volumes of poetry. The poem that is reprinted in this collection originally appeared in *two-headed woman* (University of Massachusetts Press).

Cynthia Colbert is an independent graphic designer in Lawrence, Kansas.

Activist-scholar **Angela Y. Davis's** books include *Blues Legacies and Black Feminism* (Pantheon). She is a professor in the History of Consciousness program of the University of California at Davis.

Denise Lynne Davis is a physician in private practice in Oakland, California, where she also sings and writes.

Actor and author **Ruby Dee's** works include the book written with her husband, Ossie Davis, *With Ossie and Ruby: In This Life Together* (HarperCollins), from which her piece in this anthology is taken.

Henry J. Drewal is the Evjue-Bascom Professor of Art History and Afro-American Studies at the University of Wisconsin, Madison.

Yvonne Durant is an independent writer who lives in New York City.

Thomas "Taiwo" Duvall is a musician and visual artist who lives in Clinton, Maryland.

Nikky Finney teaches in the English Department of the University of Kentucky at Lexington. She is author of *Rice* (Sister Vision) from which her poem in this anthology was reprinted.

The author of several books, **Henry Louis Gates Jr.** is chair of African-American Studies and director of the W. E. B. DuBois Center at Harvard University. His excerpt is reprinted from *Colored People* (Alfred A. Knopf).

Gloria Wade Gayles is the Rosa Mary Eminent Scholar's Chair in Humanities Fine Arts at Dillard University in New Orleans. She is the author of *Pushed Back to Strength* (Beacon Press), from which her essay in this collection was excerpted.

Jewelle Gomez is the author of six books, including the award-winning novel *The Gilda Stories*. She lives in San Francisco.

Juliette Harris is the editor of *International Review of African-American Art*, published by Hampton University Museum in Virginia. She has also written award-winning television and film documentaries.

Michael D. Harris is an assistant professor of art history at the University of North Carolina at Chapel Hill, as well as a visual artist and curator.

Peter Harris is an associate dean at Claremont College in California and the author of *Hand Me My Griot Clothes: The Autobiography of Junior Baby* (Black Classic Press).

Mark Higbee, a history professor at Eastern Michigan University, is writing a book on the politics of W. E. B. DuBois.

A professor at the City University of New York and cultural critic, **bell hooks** is the author of numerous books, including *All About Love* and the children's book on hair *Happy to Be Nappy*.

Tamara Jeffries is the health editor at *Essence* magazine.

Pamela Johnson is a former senior editor and current columnist at *Essence* magazine. She is the co-author of *Santa and Pete*, a novel published by Simon & Schuster and made into a CBS-TV movie.

Linda Jones is a feature writer for *The Dallas Morning News*.

Lisa Jones is a screenwriter and the author of *Bulletproof Diva*, from which her essay in this work was reprinted.

Mariame Kaba is a Ph.D. candidate in sociology at Northwestern University, Evanston, Ill.

Rosalie Kiah is a professor of English at Norfolk State University in Virginia.

Jacquelyn E. Long is an assistant professor of computer science at Norfolk State University.

The author of eight volumes of poetry, **Naomi Long Madgett** is the publisher-editor of Lotus Press in Detroit.

Toni Morrison is a Nobel- and Pulitzer Prize-winning author. She teaches at Princeton University. The fiction excerpt in this anthology is from her novel *Song of Solomon* (Alfred A. Knopf).

Willie Morrow is the president of California Curl and author of several works, including the seminal history *400 Years Without a Comb*.

Mark Richard Moss is an independent writer who lives in Winston-Salem, North Carolina.

Jill Nelson is the author of three books, including *Straight, No Chaser* (Penguin Putnam) from which her essay in this collection is reprinted.

Jenyne Raines is former associate beauty editor at *Essence* magazine. She lives in Brooklyn, New York.

Paitra Russell is completing her Ph.D. in anthopology at the University of Chicago.

Meg Henson Scales is a visual artist and independent writer who lives in New York City.

Ntozake Shange is the author of the Obie Award-winning play *For Colored Girls Who Have Considered Suicide/When the Rainbow Is Enuf*. She is also the author of five volumes of poetry, three novels, two children's books, and a cookbook.

S. Pearl Sharp is a filmmaker, author, and actor who lives in Los Angeles.

Leatha Simmons Mitchell is an independent writer who lives in Silver Spring, Maryland, where she dabbles in visual art and healing by way of traditional Reiki.

Laura Sullivan is a doctoral student in English at the University of Florida.

Gerrie Summers is the book and beauty editor for *Today's Black Woman* magazine and the grooming and book editor of *Black Men*. She lives in Brooklyn, New York.

Halima Taha is the author of *Collecting African American Art: Works on Paper and Canvas* (Crown Random House). An independent writer, art adviser, and appraiser, she lives in New York City.

Susan L. Taylor is a senior vice president and publication director for Essence Communications as well as a noted author and popular speaker on the lecture circuit.

Natasha Trethewey is an assistant professor of English at Auburn. She is the author of *Domestic Work* (Graywolf Press).

Alice Walker received the Pulitzer Prize in 1983 for *The Color Purple*. Her other books include *Living by the Word* (Harcourt Brace) from which her essay in this collection was taken. She resides in Northern California.

Evangeline Wheeler is associate professor of psychology at Towson State University in Maryland.

Playwright, composer, director, producer **George C. Wolfe** wrote the play *The Colored Museum*, from which his excerpt was taken. He lives in New York City.

Cherilyn ("Liv") Wright is a corporate consultant and independent writer who lives in New York City.

Toni Wynn is an independent writer who lives in Norfolk, Virginia.

Taiia Smart Young, the former new media editor of *Essence* magazine, is a city editor for an Internet company. She lives in Brooklyn, New York.